AF260890

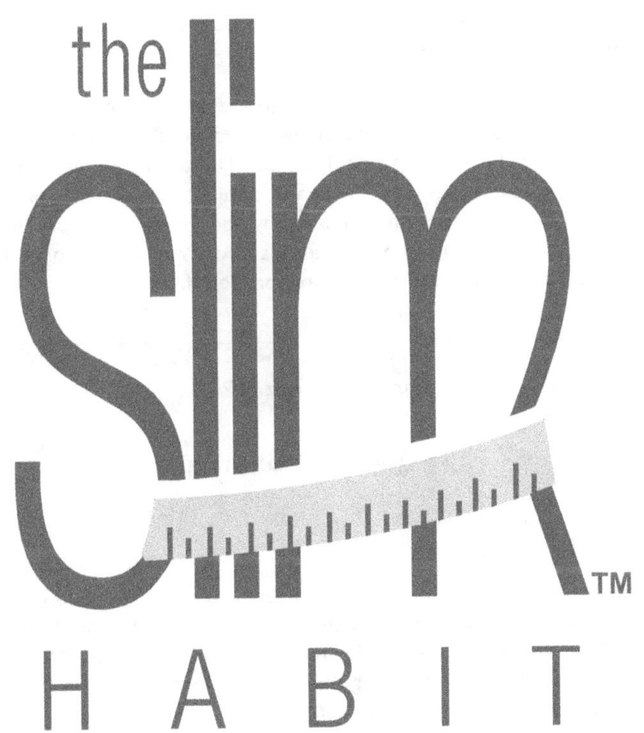
the
slim
™
HABIT

Cartoons © Roz 2020

St Quintin Publishing

The information in this book is meant to supplement, not replace, proper exercise training. All forms of exercise pose some inherent risks. The author and publisher advise readers to take full responsibility for their safety and know their limits. Before practicing the exercises in this book, be sure that your equipment is well maintained, and do not take risks beyond your level of experience, aptitude, training and fitness. The exercise programme in this book is not intended as a substitute for any exercise routine that has been prescribed by your doctor. As with all exercise programmes, you should get your doctor's approval before beginning.

ISBN 978-1-5272-0104-0

Published by St Quintin Publishing

Typeset by Mach 3 Solutions Ltd (www.mach3solutions.co.uk)

Contents

Today, it's important you do all you can to protect yourself from being seriously affected by the real and present danger that all of us face. If you are overweight or obese it's time to take the decision to lose weight. The majority of patients in intensive care units across the world have a weight problem, and their chances of survival are significantly reduced because of this.

The more fat you are carrying, the less fit you are, and the lower your lung capacity. Being overweight also means that you have a higher demand for oxygen. Your body is going to struggle to get sufficient oxygen into you blood and around your body. The consequences can be fatal.

Losing weight is more than a health choice, it's a health necessity.

By deciding to lose weight you have taken a decision that could save your life.

Introduction

Today, life has become one long feast. Unlike your hunter gatherer ancestors, you use up very little energy finding enough food to eat. There's no foraging for food, no hunting expeditions or stalking prey. All you have to do is to hunt down a supermarket, gather food from the shelves and pile your trolley high. All the food you could possibly dream of is laid out before you, and there's not a bead of sweat on your brow. The consequence of all this readily available, relatively inexpensive food is that life has become one perpetual feast. You never do without, and there's never any famine.

No famine… always available food… isn't that a good thing? Yes, of course it is. And over the past four decades the availability and choice of food and drink has increased dramatically, isn't that a good thing too? Yes… and no. Yes because we have a huge variety of delicious, tempting food to choose from, and no because too much of that food is processed food, high in sugar, salt and saturated fat. The consequences? As our food choices have increased, so has the weight of the general population, and the incidence of weight-related diseases.

If you have a weight problem you might think you know the reason why. You eat and drink too much of that delicious, tempting food, and you don't take enough exercise. This is probably true, but did you take a deliberate decision to put on weight? Was it simply greed? Did you just give into temptation, or was there something else that made you put on weight?

The truth is that if you're overweight or obese you're almost certainly NOT in control of how much you eat, or what you eat. You might think that it's you who is making the decisions, but it's not.

It's the type of food you eat and what you drink that's the problem. It can cause your body processes to malfunction to such an extent that they become the driver of your decision making, nudging your preferences towards the types of food and drink which cause you to put on weight.

What's the answer to the problem? It's not a diet. A diet is at best a sticking plaster, and doesn't address the *cause* of weight gain.

The Slim Habit approach is fundamentally different to a diet. You learn why you put on weight, how to lose it and how to maintain your weight loss. All you need is a willingness to learn, and a commitment to change.

Part One:
What you need to know

You'll discover why you put on weight. The causes are known and you have the right to know what they are. How does your body react to the food you eat? What causes it to malfunction and take control of what you eat and how much you eat? Understand why your body works against you and what the consequences are. Gain the knowledge you need to put things right, to take control of your weight and manage your weight.

Part Two:
Preparation

This is about helping you to prepare to make the changes you need to make. How to learn new habits. About raising your food awareness and how to take the right decisions about what you eat and drink. About Low Calorie Days, and why exercise is so important.

Part Three:
What to do

This is everything you need to do, your Slim Habit, set out in an easy-to-follow way. A simple, achievable programme of things to do that will deliver the outcome you want – to lose weight, to be able to manage your weight and remain slim and healthy.

Part Four:
Exercise for you

The Slim Habit guide to exercise. What type of exercise to take and how to get the best out of exercise. It includes useful tips and illustrations.

The Slim Habit is a new, fresh approach to losing weight, managing your weight and staying slim and healthy. This is *your* Slim Habit, your opportunity for a better life.

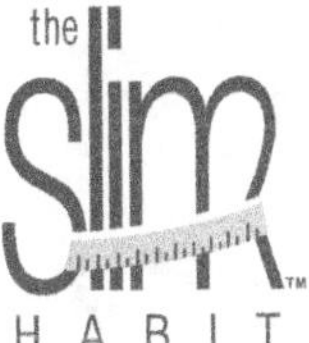

Part One

What You Need To Know

If you've tried to lose weight you know what an uphill struggle it can be. If you've been on a diet and the weight has returned, as it inevitably does, it's very dispiriting. When it comes to losing weight and getting healthy, there are better things to do than going on a diet.

The good news is that there's new, fresh thinking about why you put on weight, about how your body reacts to the modern diet and how it affects your weight and your health. If you understand why things happen, the reasons *why* you put on weight, you can make changes that will revolutionise your life. With the help of The Slim Habit, you *can* lose weight and not put it back on again, and you *can* manage and control your weight. It doesn't involve a restrictive regime like a diet, just the application of knowledge, a commitment to make change and common sense.

But first, let's start by asking some fundamental questions …

If you're overweight or obese, do you think it's fair you should get all the blame? Do you really think it's your fault, your responsibility? Did you make a deliberate choice to put on weight? It's very easy for people to point fingers, isn't it? Very easy to accuse … greedy, no sense of responsibility, self-indulgent, no self-control …

Whoa! These accusations are both unfair and wrong!

Do we eat too much? Yes we do. Do we take too little exercise? Yes we do. Is this why we are getting fatter? Yes it is. **BUT!** The real question that needs to be asked is: What's the *reason* behind our seemingly insatiable appetite and our ever-expanding waistline?

In the last 30 years obesity rates have trebled. In the case of adolescents it has quadrupled. Can this be simply down to greed, a lack of responsibility, self-indulgence, no self-control? **Absolutely not!**

So where does the blame lie?

Despite protestations of innocence from the food industry, **it IS what you eat and drink that's the root cause of your weight gain**. Why? Because your body just can't cope with the concentration of calorie-dense, low-fibre ingredients contained in the modern diet.

We eat *a lot* of processed food. Much of it contains high levels of sugar, salt, saturated fat – and very little fibre. Too much of what we drink contains excessive amounts of sugar or sweeteners. The reality is that the food you eat messes with your biochemistry *so much* that it takes over. You lose control of what you eat – and how much you eat.

What's your biochemistry?

Biochemical reactions go on in your body all the time; they're a network of chemical processes that maintain and regulate your life. Chemical processes that keep you 'in sync and in tune'. When you eat lots of processed food, and drink large quantities of sugary drinks, it plays havoc with these chemical processes. It puts a spanner in your works – and *you* don't work. Your system breaks down, your finely-tuned chemical processes are turned on their head, and they malfunction in such a way that **your biochemistry becomes the driver of what and how much you eat, not you.**

So what's happened?

The cause of this malfunction is actually quite simple. It's happened because of **a mismatch between what you eat and drink and your body's ability to process it**. It's this mismatch that is the root cause of weight gain, a mismatch that all too often also leads to ill health. The truth is that you were not designed to eat large quantities of low-fibre, calorie-dense, sugary, salty, fatty food – or to drink litres of sugar-laced sodas, fruit juice or smoothies.

This mismatch has its roots in the past. It's actually an **evolutionary mismatch.** You see …

You can't ignore your evolutionary past!

The evolutionary mismatch – what it means.

In evolutionary terms, your body has not had time to adapt to the modern diet. It is still programmed to deal with the life of your hunter gatherer ancestors, who led a tough life. They spent most of their time looking for food and coping with feast and famine. However, over thousands of years their bodies evolved to be able to cope with this.

It's easy to forget that it's only 5,000 years since the development of agriculture and animal husbandry was established. In evolutionary terms that's the blink of an eye. The industrialisation of food started a mere 200 years ago. Today we don't have to spend time and energy foraging for our food or dealing with famine. For most of us food is abundant and relatively inexpensive.

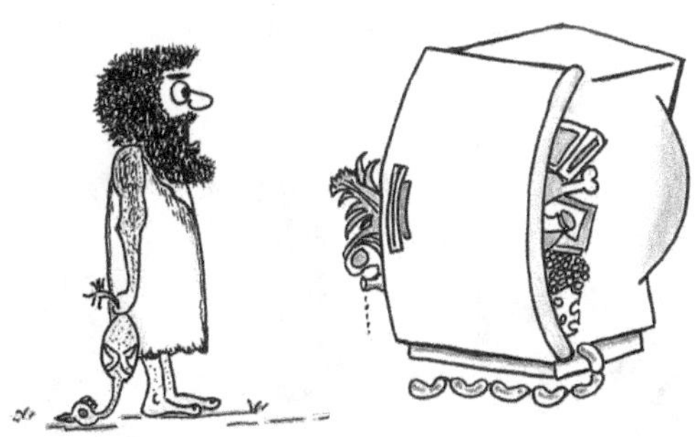

The problem we face now is that not enough time has passed to allow our bodies to evolve from being active hunter gatherers who survived on a sugar-free diet which was high in fibre, to sedentary beings gorging on a calorie-dense diet of processed foods, high in sugar and low in fibre.

Our biological evolution has not kept pace with our cultural evolution

The consequence is a mismatch between the food our bodies have evolved to deal with, and the type of food we eat today, which our bodies find difficult to process.

The effect of this mismatch is a malfunction of our biochemical processes which results in weight gain – and which eventually can lead to weight-related diseases such as diabetes, heart disease, stroke and certain types of cancer.

Where have we gone wrong?

There has been a failure to understand that it is an evolutionary mismatch which is the root cause of our inability to control our weight, and the main cause of the increase in weight-related diseases.

Distracted by a confusion of diet advice, and by diets that claim to have the definitive answer to weight loss, the evidence of an evolutionary mismatch has been overlooked.

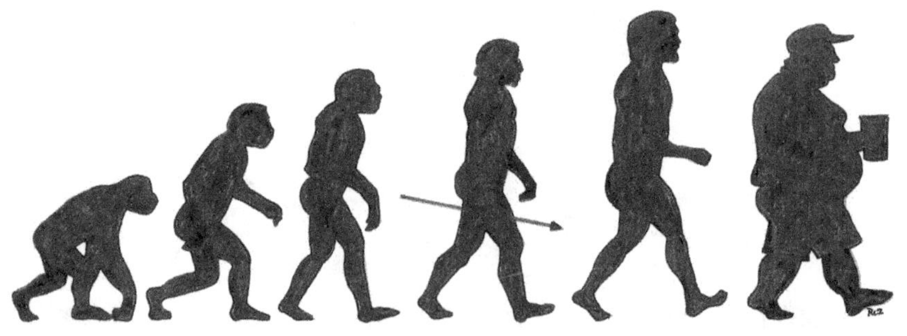

Time to face up to reality

Unlike our ancestors, our modern lifestyle is one perpetual feast, a feast of processed food and drink, high in sugar and low in fibre. There is never any famine, never any time when we don't have access to food. This affects the amount of exercise we take. We don't take enough exercise because the prime motivation **to move**, to find food, no longer exits.

By subjecting our bodies to an avalanche of processed food and drink, and by depriving it of enough necessary exercise, we have created a modern-day phenomenon, an evolutionary mismatch which is *the* cause of so many people being overweight – and a worldwide obesity epidemic.

And there are other contributory factors …

The **stress** of modern day life, of trying your best to cope with all the demands and pressures that life throws at you, of being overweight or obese, takes its toll. What happens when you're under stress? Your body reacts by producing the stress hormone cortisol. The problem with cortisol is that frequent exposure to this hormone drives weight gain.

And then there's **temptation**. Those constant reminders about food and drink. Advertisements on TV encouraging you to snack, snack, snack. Magazines and billboards, with images of mouth-watering meals. Fast-food outlets on every street corner pushing their bargain burgers, and supermarket shelves crammed with delicious food. You are surrounded by prompts to eat. The temptation is to keep eating.

All this pressure to consume – driven by profit-hungry food companies and supermarkets – has had a dramatic effect on your eating habits. You not only eat at mealtimes, **you are persuaded to eat – to snack – all through the day**. There's hardly a time when you're not chewing or drinking. You never give your body a rest. *It's always processing food.* It never has time to rest and restore itself.

And then the consequences …

All these things have consequences. Weight gain, yes – and a strong possibility you will be plagued by the diseases that result from being overweight or obese, such as type 2 diabetes, high blood pressure, heart attack, stroke, dementia and cancer. And to add to your cheer, you age more quickly and you die before your time.

If your weight and health are being compromised by an evolutionary mismatch, isn't it time to find out what you can do about it? Time to **get wise, time to get yourself in sync** with your evolutionary present?

If you want to be in control of your weight and lead an active, healthy life, **your diet and your lifestyle have to be in sync** with the way your system, your body, works. **You can't fast forward the evolutionary clock**. You have to respect where it is in biological terms. If you are to avoid being overweight or obese, you have to align your eating habits and your lifestyle to be compatible with where you are in your evolutionary development if you want to live a long and healthy life.

Knowledge is everything …

If you know why things happen, how your body works, how it reacts to certain foods, you'll understand why your biochemistry has become the driver of what and how much you eat and drink. The greater your knowledge, the easier it will be for you to take back control and make change.

It's not difficult to understand …

The human body *is* complicated, but the explanations here have been simplified to make it easy to understand.

Let's make a start …

Let's begin with your metabolism. What is it?

It's the process of breaking down food and turning it into energy.

Why do you need to know about it?

Because how your body processes food, and how your body reacts to the food you eat is the key to everything.

Okay, but how does it work? What does your body do with what you eat? What effect does what you eat have on you? And crucially, what drives you to eat?

It all starts with motivation!

You have two prime motivators, ***hunger* and *reward***.

Let's look at **hunger** first.

Motivator Number 1: Hunger

Why do you eat? You eat food because it gives you the energy you need to function, and the vitamins and minerals you need to maintain your body. Food contains calories which you metabolise and use to build muscle and bone – and to produce energy.

The food that you eat is a mixture of fat, protein, carbohydrate and fibre.

When you chew and then swallow food (calories) you start an amazing process. Here's what happens:

The process

The food you eat first passes into your stomach where hydrochloric acid is released. This breaks the food down into smaller pieces before it passes through into your small intestine, where digestive juices (enzymes) digest the food into even smaller pieces.

The digestive juices in your small intestine break down your food into three nutrients: fatty acids, amino acids and simple sugars.

Nutrients are the essential substances we get from the food we eat. They provide energy and supply the body with all it needs to perform its daily functions properly.

Dietary fats are broken down into **fatty acids**, dietary proteins into **amino acids** and carbohydrates into **simple sugars** – which is mostly glucose. Your small intestine's job is to absorb these nutrients and send them to your liver for them to be processed into energy. Any **fibre** in your food is not digested. Instead, fibre does two things: it speeds the flow of food through your intestine and, importantly, **it limits the rate of absorption of the three nutrients.** More about the benefits of fibre later.

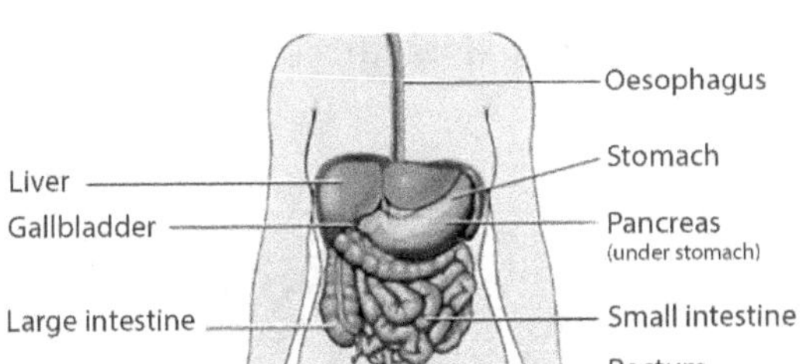

When the nutrients arrive at your liver, its job is to process them and turn them into energy. This causes a rise in your blood glucose level. The rise in blood glucose is picked up by your **pancreas** which prompts it to release a hormone called **insulin.**

*Your pancreas is a very important organ which sits behind your stomach. It delivers digestive juices into your small intestine which helps to digest your food. It's also responsible for releasing the hormone **insulin** into your bloodstream.*

What is insulin? Insulin is most commonly known as the hormone that regulates blood sugar. Blood glucose is produced when your liver processes the nutrients it receives from your digestive tract – your small intestine. Your pancreas then releases just the right amount of insulin to match the level of glucose in your blood to ensure your blood glucose level is kept in balance: not too high, not too low.

Insulin is also your energy storage hormone. It takes the glucose from your blood and stores it for future use as glycogen. Some of it goes to your liver, some to your muscles. Then it takes the fatty acids in your blood and turns them into triglycerides (fat) and stuffs them into your fat cells for future long-term use. Insulin is your energy parking attendant, if you like – a very clever parking attendant. Once fat has been stored in your fat cells, your parking attendant guards them and won't allow any release until your other energy stores are running low. When your insulin levels drop, when you need energy, only then will fatty acids be released into your blood stream. They will then be burned by your liver and other organs to give you the energy you need.

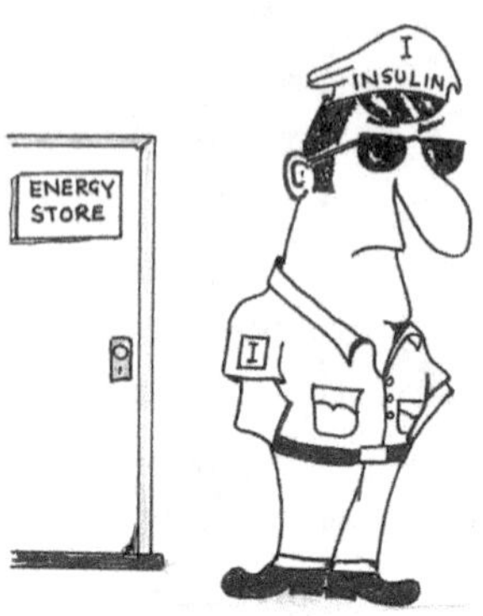

How does your body keep your energy in balance?

You need a constant supply of energy to carry out routine tasks, but you also need energy reserves for emergencies. So, balancing your energy needs: what you need, how much you need and how much you need to store, is very important. How is this done?

At the base of your brain there's a small, very important area called the **hypothalamus**. It's about the size of a pea. This tiny part of your brain controls many hormonal systems in your body. Importantly, it controls your energy balance. You could call it your energy balance supervisor.

So, what *is* energy balance? **Energy balance is the relationship between 'energy in', the calories you consume, and 'energy out', the energy you use.** You don't want to run out of energy because then you wouldn't be able to function properly. You need enough energy to be available to meet your needs. Your energy has to be kept in balance.

In order to control this balance, your hypothalamus needs information on your energy status. It gets this from organs in your body via hormones circulating in your bloodstream. It is always aware of how much energy you are using, and how much you have stored.

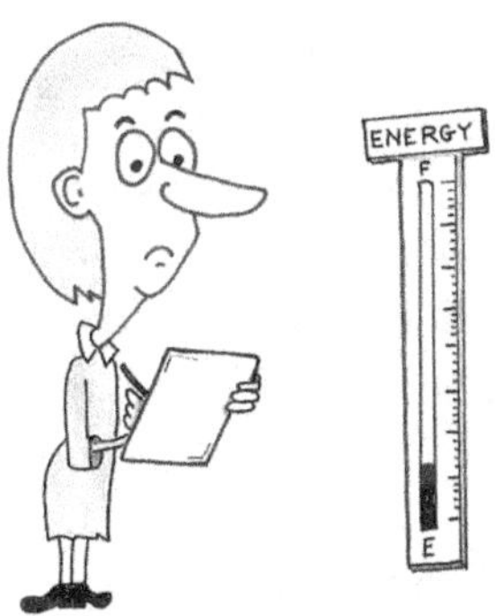

The feedback to the hypothalamus, your energy supervisor, is constant. It has to be if your energy balance is to be maintained. It's always busy gathering information and then sending out instructions. This happens via your pituitary gland, often called your 'master gland' because it controls several other glands in your body.

Your hypothalamus has other sources of information too. An important source is your **vagus nerve** because it connects your brain to your liver, your intestines, your pancreas, and your fat cells. It's a huge source of information on your energy storage status, and acts as an information super-highway between your brain and your organs – and vice versa. It communicates information from your stomach that you feel hungry via your hunger hormone ghrelin, as well as vital information from your liver when it is processing nutrients during a meal. It informs your hypothalamus whether you need more food or you don't, and communicates when you are full from a hormone called PYY, which is released in your small intestine.

There's also a small, but extremely important part of the hypothalamus, called the **Ventromedial Hypothalamus** or **VMH** – let's call it the supervisor's assistant. It's also in the energy storage and management business. It controls energy storage and consumption. It always wants to know how hungry you are or how full you are. It gets this information from your gastro-intestinal tract – from your stomach and your intestines . It also gathers long-term information on the state of your fat stores: how much energy you have stored away for a rainy day, and whether you need to eat more calories to keep your energy stores topped up. It's constantly got its eye on your fuel gauge. This vital information is delivered by the hormones leptin and insulin. The **VMH then uses all this information to either stimulate or suppress your appetite.**

How is your energy storage managed?

Balancing your energy needs is one thing, but how is it managed? A key piece of information your **hypothalamus** needs to know is **how much energy you have stored in your fat cells**. Is the amount of energy you have stored okay? How much fuel do you have in your tank? How does it get this information? It gets it from a hormone called **leptin**. Leptin is produced by your fat cells and circulates in your bloodstream. We all have our own energy storage level which is the amount sufficient to meet our particular needs. The level of leptin indicates whether the energy you have stored is above or below that level.

In signalling whether your energy level is above or below your normal level, leptin sends out one of two messages. *"I'm not hungry. I have energy to burn "* (anorexigenesis) or *"I'm hungry. My energy stores are low"* (orexigenesis) Your hypothalamus is *always* on the lookout for leptin signals. It's constantly evaluating them to keep your energy in balance.

So, it's very important for your **VMH**, your hypothalamus's assistant whose business it is to control energy storage and consumption, to pick up information from your leptin signals.

When it reads that you have enough energy, and there is enough energy stored, your hypothalamus tells your sympathetic nervous system, which is responsible for fat loss, **to turn *on***. *"I'm ready for action and I have plenty of stored energy"*. It also turns *off* the vagus nerve **which is responsible for stimulating your appetite and for fat gain**. *"I'm not hungry and I don't need to store any energy"*.

If your **VMH** reads from your leptin signals that your energy levels are low**, it turns *off*** your sympathetic nervous system because you are low on energy and need to store fat. *"My energy level is low. I need to save energy"* and it turns ***on*** your vagus nerve, which communicates the feeling of hunger between your stomach and your brain. This stimulates your appetite and promotes fat storage. *"I'm hungry, my energy reserves are low and I need to store energy. Please I need to eat more food, and store more fat."*

*If you've been on a diet you'll have experienced this. When you go on a diet you reduce your food intake and your fat cells lose fat. Your energy storage level drops below your normal level. This means you produce **less leptin**. So the message your VMH picks up is that your energy storage level is below normal. Guess what? You feel hungry, you obey and you go in search of something to eat. Easy to see why diets don't work! When you diet your body actually **works against** your efforts to lose weight.*

The crucial role of leptin

Leptin is produced by your fat cells to provide information on the state of your fat stores. **Leptin** is a vital hormone in your energy management process. It's not only the provider of information to your **VMH**, it also has a crucial role in ensuring your energy needs are kept in balance.

Now this is where it all starts to go wrong!

What happens if your VMH fails to pick up any leptin signals?

Your **VMH**, always on the alert, is constantly looking for leptin signals. This is because its Number One concern is to manage your energy needs to ensure your survival. If it can't pick up any leptin signals, and has no information to guide it, it thinks the worst. **It thinks you're starving.**

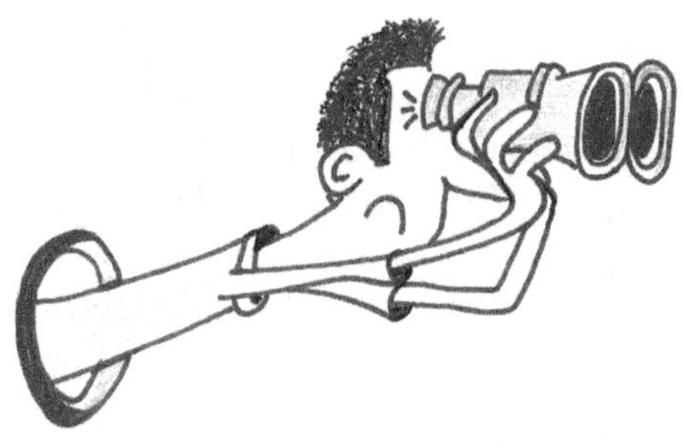

Leptin…leptin…I see no leptin…

So what does it do? It automatically reverts to its default setting. **It gets you to store energy**. To do this it signals to your sympathetic nervous system that you need to reduce activity in order to conserve energy. The effect of this is to make you feel tired and listless. All you feel like doing is sitting on the sofa and watching TV.

But it doesn't stop there. Desperate to find those missing leptin signals so that it can understand what to do, your VMH sends an emergency signal to the vagus nerve to tell your pancreas to **release more insulin.** Producing excess insulin is its remedy. It forces your pancreas to produce more insulin in the hope that, by doing so, it will to get you to make leptin and it will then get the information it needs.

But more insulin doesn't work. It still can't make out any leptin signals. The result is that you end up with far too much insulin in your system. **You go on eating**, and insulin goes about its business of storing fat. Your fat cells get stuffed with more and more fat. **The more insulin, the more fat is stored.** You suffer non-stop energy storage – and you put on weight, lots of it.

When this happens, when your VMH can't pick up any leptin signals, you are what is called **"leptin resistant"**.

What causes leptin resistance? Insulin!

It's too much insulin that triggers leptin resistance. It's insulin that blocks vital leptin signals, so your VMH is blind to those vital signals which would tell it you're full, that you need to stop eating – which of course you don't, and so the weight piles on.

What causes your pancreas to produce so much insulin?

Too much low-fibre processed food, high in sugar and saturated fat – and sugary drinks! *This* is the cause of your evolutionary mismatch. *This* is what causes your biochemistry to get turned on its head!

So what effect does all this insulin have?

Remember, insulin is your energy storage hormone. So **the more insulin you produce, the more fat is stuffed into your fat cells**. However, the worst effect of lots of insulin in your system is that you become **insulin resistant.**

What is insulin resistance?

Insulin resistance means that the ability of your cells to respond to insulin is diminished. Your cells become resistant, desensitised to the effects of insulin. This means that insulin, your energy storage hormone, is unable to store energy properly or to control the level of glucose in your body.

So what happens?

Imagine insulin knocking at the door of your muscle cells. It needs to store energy. *"Let me in, I've got energy for you to store"*. In normal circumstances the door would be opened and the energy would be allowed in. When you become insulin resistant, the door remains closed. Your muscle can't hear the knock: it's 'resistant', deaf to the knocking. When there is no response to the knock, your pancreas responds **by making more insulin** to make the knock louder. But the door remains closed, and as a result your blood glucose levels rise.

However, your fat cells are different, they're not quite so deaf, they **can** hear the knocking. Unlike your muscle cells, your fat cells retain most of their sensitivity. As a result, insulin puts the energy in the only place it can find that will open its door. **It stuffs it into your fat cells.**

And the blame for all this lies with …low-fibre processed food high in sugar and saturated fat – and those sugar laden drinks.

It's the type of food and how much of it you eat that's the problem.

If you are always eating an energy-dense, high-sugar, low-fibre processed food diet, and drinking sugary beverages, your liver will be constantly overwhelmed by an avalanche of nutrients, and your pancreas will be forever producing insulin. With so much insulin being produced you will eventually become insulin resistant. As a consequence you put on weight, lots of it.

Insulin resistance – this is when the evolutionary mismatch really hits home!

Fibre: Why It's So Important

What is fibre? Dietary fibre is found in vegetables, fruit, peas, beans and whole grains. You can't digest fibre, you derive no energy from it, yet it's a very important part of a healthy diet.

There are two types of fibre, **soluble and insoluble.**

Soluble fibre absorbs water and, vitally, it slows down the rate of absorption of food in the gut. Examples of soluble fibre are peas, beans, lentils, fruit and vegetables. **Insoluble fibre** doesn't dissolve in water and helps to speed the passage of food through your gut. They are the tough, hard-to-chew part of grains and fruit. Other examples of insoluble fibre are: whole grains and wheat bran, beans such as kidney beans, green leafy vegetables, nuts and seeds.

Low fibre and insulin.

The fact that processed food contains low levels of fibre has a significant impact on the amount of insulin your pancreas produces.

It's your small intestine's job to absorb nutrients from the food you eat and send them to your liver so they can be processed into energy.

When you eat food containing fibre, the fibre forms a gel-like glutinous barrier between the food and the wall of your small intestine. This has the effect of **slowing down the rate that nutrients from your food are absorbed and sent to your liver.** Consequently your liver receives a steady flow of nutrients which it processes gradually. Your pancreas is able to keep your blood glucose at the right level and to release just the right amount of insulin to store the new energy in the right place, efficiently and effectively.

When there is very little fibre in your diet …

When you eat high-calorie, energy-dense processed food which contains very little fibre, no glutinous barrier is produced to slow down the absorption of nutrients. This causes the nutrients in your small intestine to be absorbed **very quickly** because there is nothing to slow the process down. The result is that **an avalanche of nutrients** is dumped on your liver. As a result your blood glucose levels rise sharply, and **your pancreas produces lots of insulin to deal with the problem.**

And you thought you could trust branded food …

Food companies deliberately remove fibre from the processed foods they manufacture. Why? Because fibre reduces shelf life and fibre doesn't freeze well. This is the reason why frozen ready meals and fast foods contain very low levels of fibre.

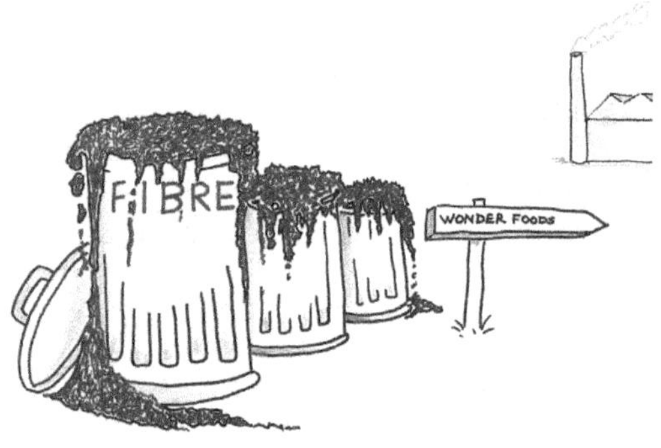

Again – it's the low-fibre processed food you eat that messes with your biochemistry

Today the average person eats less than 15 grams of fibre a day. Your ancestors used to eat more than 100 grams. They may have had many problems to contend with, but being overweight was not one of them! **You should eat a minimum of 30 grams of fibre a day.**

Sugar – Public Enemy Number One!

In your evolutionary past you would have consumed hardly any sugar. It was difficult to get, and eaten very rarely. Today sugar is everywhere and in practically everything. We eat huge amounts of it. Sugar consumption has tripled in the last thirty years. And guess what? The rise in the consumption of sugar has gone hand-in-hand with the rise in the levels of obesity. No coincidence.

We consume between 100 and 130 pounds of sugar every year and most of the sugar we eat comes from calorie-dense, low-fibre, processed food and sugary drinks.

So what's wrong with sugar? The simple answer is nothing – in small doses. It's the **quantity** of sugar we consume that's the problem. Here's why:

Sugar (or sucrose), is made up of 50% glucose and 50% fructose. It's a carbohydrate, a simple carbohydrate, but it has a unique quality. It's unique because its constituent parts, glucose and fructose, are metabolised differently. Glucose can be metabolised, (processed into energy), by all your organs, with only about 20% being metabolised by your liver. Fructose on the other hand is different. It is *almost completely metabolised by your liver*. And this is the root of the problem. Why? Because your liver turns fructose into free fatty acids, then into triglycerides, which get stored as fat. **Fructose is metabolised as fat.**

A diet high in sugar is a **high fat** diet.

Beware of all products that contain fructose and particularly High Fructose Corn Syrup (HFCS). **Fructose makes you fat.**

Be wary of products labelled 'low fat'. They may not be quite what they seem. They may have a reduced fat content, but the fat has been replaced by ...**sugar**! Why? Because reducing fat content makes processed food taste bland. Adding sugar solves the problem and makes the food taste more palatable.

So beware! Low fat can mean high fat because fat has been substituted by sugar.

Sugar in excess is a toxin!

In the quantities sugar is being consumed today, it is a toxin. Here's are some reasons why ...

1. When you consume fructose either as sugar or as high fructose corn syrup (HFCS), it doesn't stimulate an insulin response. The result? Your leptin level doesn't rise. Your hypothalamus isn't aware your energy stores are full ...and **you keep eating**.

2. When you're hungry, the cells in your stomach produce a hormone called ghrelin. This is your hunger signal. When you eat glucose it suppresses ghrelin and you begin to feel less hungry. When you eat fructose it does the opposite. It doesn't suppress ghrelin. **You continue to feel hungry, and you keep eating.**

3. When there's too much fructose in your diet there is a good chance that, over time, it will damage your liver. This can lead to insulin liver resistance. When this happens your pancreas generates higher levels of insulin. **More insulin, more fat**. This leads to two other things:
   a) Leptin resistance – this prevents your hypothalamus from seeing any leptin signals, and when this happens it thinks you're starving, and **you keep eating.**
   b) It also affects your reward system. The consequence is **a vicious cycle of continuous consumption**, which can

eventually lead to disease, to metabolic syndrome. More on your reward system later.

(Metabolic syndrome is a group of risk factors which include obesity, diabetes, lipid problems, high blood pressure and cardio-vascular disease.)

4. The fat cells that fill up most from fructose consumption are visceral fat cells. Fructose is very efficient at building up toxic, pro-inflammatory visceral fat. This is the bad fat that collects round your internal organs, and also manifests itself as belly fat. **Visceral fat is dangerous fat**. It secretes pro-inflammatory hormones into your bloodstream which can lead to the increased risk of diseases such as cardiovascular disease, type 2 diabetes and cancer.

5. It was never intended that we **drink** our calories. **Today we drink in excess of 25% of our calories**. This is usually through sugary drinks, fruit juice and smoothies. The problem is that liquid sugar calories, glucose, fructose, and particularly high fructose corn syrup (HCFS), **are not registered by the brain** as food, so you don't compensate by eating less.

The food we eat has been contaminated by too much sugar.

Successful long-term weight loss and better health has to come from an 'eyes wide open' new relationship with sugar and the products that contain too much of it. Why? There are two reasons. First because sugar is addictive. Sugar ticks all the boxes of an addictive substance. Secondly, because the amount of sugar we are eating is, slowly but surely, killing us.

*The World health Organisation recommends your RDA (Recommended Daily Allowance) for sugar should be **25 grams**.*

Now you know!

Now you know that what you eat and drink can seriously affect your biochemistry. **The ultimate consequence of a diet that causes your biochemistry to malfunction is insulin resistance**. It's the marker of a complete mismatch with your evolutionary present. Until you change your diet and your lifestyle, your biochemistry will continue to drive your behaviour, not you. You will continue to put on weight.

Oh, and there's something else you need to know…

In our desperation to reduce or control our weight we have become obsessed with calories without understanding that…

A calorie is not a calorie!

The food industry would have you believe that all calories are the same. They're not …

All calories release the same amount of energy. But a calorie is a measurement of energy, it's not a measurement of nutritional value, nor is it an indicator of how your body uses the energy you get from different foods.

Despite the spin from the food industry, a calorie is not a calorie as far as your body is concerned. Treating all calories as equal is a huge mistake, but a convenient one if your purpose is to disguise the effect of your processed products on people, and shift the blame for what they do to you to the decisions *you* make.

The fact is that your body deals with carbohydrates, proteins and fats in very different ways. They don't go through the same biochemical pathways and each one has different effects. Each has a huge influence on the biological processes that govern what, when, and how much you eat.

Take carbohydrates for example. There are two classes of carbohydrate, sugar and starch. Starch is made up of glucose only, but sugar is made up of glucose **and** fructose. While glucose can be metabolised by all the organs in your body, the bulk of fructose can only be metabolised by your liver – as fat. Even although glucose and fructose have the same chemical formula, fructose has more effect on your biochemistry, much of it detrimental. It also affects your appetite and your metabolic health. **A calorie is not a calorie.**

Fat? Not all fats are the same. There are good fats and bad fats. Good fats have valuable anti-inflammatory properties, bad fats can promote weight related diseases. **A calorie is not a calorie**.

When it comes to protein, your body is less efficient at metabolising it. It takes much more energy to metabolise protein than it does carbohydrate or fat. The effect is that it reduces your appetite. Protein calories are less fattening than carbohydrate or fat calories. **A calorie is not a calorie.**

A calorie is definitely not a calorie! Different sources of calories do very different things. They affect your biochemistry is very different ways.

It's the type and quality of the processed food you eat and drink that's important. How it affects your biochemistry determines how much you eat, how much you weigh and the state of your health.

So…

What you eat has given you a problem that your body can't solve, but *you* can. With the Slim Habit you *can* make changes in your life to regain control, and get in sync with your evolutionary present.

Now let's look at your second prime motivator …

Motivator Number Two – Reward

We all have an ingenious system hard-wired in us. Sometimes called our 'master motivator', it's our **reward system**. It's an extremely smart mechanism we all possess which plays a vital role in our lives.

Why a reward system?

Think about it. If there was no element of reward in your life, you wouldn't be motivated to do much. Why would you do something unless there was some benefit in it for you? On the other hand if you are rewarded for doing something, you have motivation. If you didn't enjoy sex you wouldn't do it. So reward has a vital role in the perpetuation of the human race. If you didn't enjoy eating you would be reluctant to spend time looking for nutritious things to eat, and you would fatally compromise your ability to survive.

It's easy to see why reward plays an important part in your survival. Over thousands of years our reward mechanism has developed to be the force that drives what we do, what we need to do. Whether you like it or not, you are programmed to seek out things that give you pleasure, that reward you.

So how does your reward system work?

There's a 'pathway' in your brain, a neurochemical pathway, sometimes called the hedonic pathway, a pathway to pleasure, if you like. It is a communication channel from a part of your brain called the ventral tagmental area or **VTA** to your nucleus accumbens – we'll call this **Reward Central.**

When you eat something tasty, this alerts your VTA and triggers it to send a signal to Reward Central to release dopamine. The result is that you experience a feeling of pleasure.

So what is dopamine? Dopamine is a neurotransmitter. A neurotransmitter is something that signals between one part of your brain and another. In the case of dopamine, between your **VTA** and **Reward Central**. When dopamine is released it produces a feeling of pleasure.

This pleasurable feeling is a **reward**. A reward for eating, for supplying your body with food that it can convert into energy. A reward for doing the right thing to ensure your survival.

Once you have had enough to eat, the feeling of pleasure subsides. Your VTA receives a signal to stop releasing dopamine and you stop eating. Where does this signal come from? It comes from **leptin**. Remember leptin, the messenger from your fat cells who says you have enough energy and you don't need any more food? **Leptin switches off reward.** The motivation to eat disappears.

Insulin also has a role to play. The rise in insulin, which happens when you eat, also helps to blunt the feeling of reward. You no longer feel the need to continue eating. This is an important safety mechanism because it allows you to enjoy a slice of chocolate cake and really enjoy it, but stops you from eating the whole cake. You can see that both leptin and insulin are important regulators of your reward system.

But what happens if you're insulin resistant?

This is where the problems begin. If you're insulin resistant because of the effect of all that processed food and those sugar-laced sodas you've consumed, then **your VTA will be resistant to leptin**. It won't see any leptin signals telling it to stop releasing dopamine. Also, insulin won't clear down dopamine from **reward central**. The consequence of this is disastrous.

If the release of dopamine isn't stopped, if dopamine keeps on being released, you keep on being rewarded for eating. The feeling of pleasure continues. You keep eating.

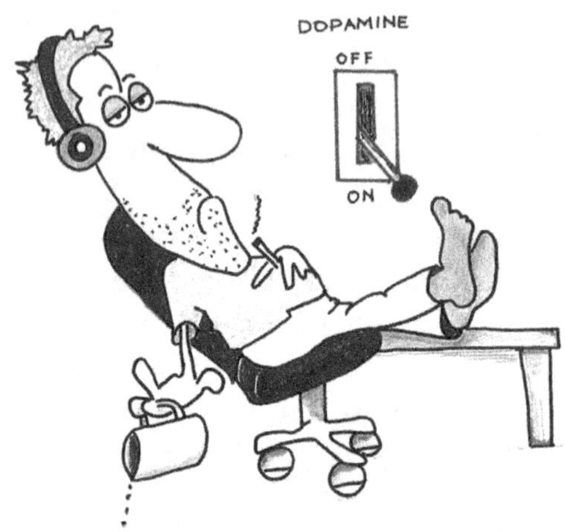

Meanwhile at Reward Central no messages had been received

This happens despite the fact that your energy stores are full. Meanwhile your trusty energy storage hormone insulin keeps doing its job. You keep eating, it keeps on stuffing your fat cells with fat. And so starts a vicious cycle of continuous consumption and weight gain.

Unfortunately, there's a double whammy. Why? Because **sweet things** hit the spot. They give you the greatest pleasure. You crave the very things you need to avoid: cookies, cakes and candy, all full of the demon sugar.

But What About Sweeteners?

Sweeteners contain few, if any, calories. They occur in many processed foods, in sodas and juices, so are they bad for you too or are they a good substitute for sugar? If sugar is public enemy number one, are sweetners the answer, and how does your body react to sweeteners?

When sweeteners were first introduced they were deemed to be a safe, 'no calorie' option to sugar. 'Sugar Free' and 'Diet' products containing sweeteners such as saccharine and aspartame appeared everywhere. But following years of research, sweeteners now appear not to be the wonder ingredient they were once heralded to be.

Sweetners may reduce your sugar consumption, but they may also make you *put on* weight, not lose it.

Why? Because when you eat or drink something containing a sweetener your brain is tricked into believing that something pleasurable containing calories is going to arrive – like sugar.

As soon as you taste the sweetness of the sweetener, your reward system is activated just as it would be with sugar, and dopamine is released. This where the problems start. Because the sweetener contains no calories, there's nothing to activate leptin, nothing to switch off your reward system. Nothing to stop the release of dopamine. The result is that you don't want the good feeling to stop so you continue to drink more sweetened soda.

But here's the rub! When no calories appear, your brain feels cheated. It wants to make up for the calories it's been cheated out of. As a consequence you go looking for something make up for all those missing calories, and your preference is usually a sugary snack. The result is that you end up eating more calories than you might otherwise have done, and you put on weight.

Drinks containing sweeteners, artificial ones like saccharine and aspartame or natural sweeteners such as Stevia and derivatives, are **NOT** the answer to the sugar problem. All they do is create another problem which has the same outcome – weight gain!

Diet drinks should not be part of your diet!

In addition, there is new evidence that artificial sweeteners disrupt microflora (essential bacteria, microscopic algae and fungi) in your gut. These microflora are very important for your general health. When they are disrupted they drive glucose intolerance which increases your chances of becoming obese and of developing type 2 diabetes.

Sweeteners have been around for a long time. If sweeteners were the wonder substitute for sugar they claim to be there would have been something to show for it, a reduction in weight in the general population, for example. There has been no such reduction – in fact there has been a significant increase.

Beware! Food companies are coming under increasing pressure to reduce the sugar content in sodas. Sugar *will be* replaced by sweeteners. This might reduce your sugar consumption, but have absolutely no effect on your weight – except that it might increase!

It's your diet – again!

The evolutionary mismatch strikes again. The effect of your energy-dense, high-in-sugar, low-in-fibre processed food diet, and all those sugary drinks are to blame. Your compromised biochemistry now plays havoc with your reward system.

And then, on top of everything else, 'life' works against you!

Stress

Everybody experiences stress in their daily lives, but what is stress? Stress can be positive, a motivator even. It can keep you sharp and aware, but when you suffer too much stress, it's bad for you. Recent studies have found that there's a link between increased levels of stress and being overweight or obese. So it's important to know why this link occurs and how to deal with it.

What stress does

Your body has a response to stress. Whenever you experience stress, real or imagined, your brain interprets it as a threat. This response is very much a part of our evolutionary history, when survival depended upon an immediate reaction to a threat, when the options open to you were either to 'fight or take flight'. Whatever option you chose required lots of instant energy. Today, the circumstances which threaten us, which cause us stress, may not be life-threatening, but your brain reacts in the same way as it did thousands of years ago.

Here's what happens …

When you're stressed, your amygdala, which is part of your emotional brain, signals to your hypothalamus that you are under stress. It then alerts your 'master gland', your pituitary gland, to tell your adrenal glands (they sit on top of your kidneys) to release a hormone called **cortisol.**

What does cortisol do and how does it work?

Cortisol is an amazing hormone. It has the effect of switching you into a different gear. It ups the ante and helps you to cope with the threat, the stress you feel. What does it do?

When cortisol enters your bloodstream, it immediately shuts down anything that can't help you deal with the 'threat'. It focuses your brain and reduces your cells' responsiveness to insulin, so that energy storage stops. This immediately prompts your cells to switch from storing energy to supplying energy. Your blood glucose levels then rise, allowing you instant access to energy. It also increases your heart rate, and your blood pressure rises too. You are ready for action.

And then …

After the threat has passed and your stress level falls, cortisol is switched off …at least that's what *should* happen.

How cortisol affects us today

It's easy to see how useful cortisol was in our evolutionary past. The threats we experienced were immediate and probably life-threatening. Today, cortisol is activated not by the threat posed by a sabre-toothed tiger, but by the stresses we experience in everyday life – and there are many. A bullying boss, financial worries, relationship problems, the pressure of work, bringing up small children, paying the mortgage, weight worries. It's a long list.

The problem is that the stresses we experience today tend not to be the momentary threats we experienced in our evolutionary past. They can be **constant and unrelenting**. This means that our stress response can remain active for very long periods. Cortisol hangs around. Long-term exposure to too much cortisol is not good for you, and plays a big part in weight gain.

The effect of too much stress – and too much cortisol

When you become stressed the immediate effect of cortisol is to dampen your appetite, but this only lasts for a short time, a matter of minutes. **As cortisol levels rise, your appetite increases.** In evolutionary terms, the purpose of this was to shut down your appetite while you dealt with the threat, and then increase it to replenish the energy reserves you used up dealing with the threat.

In today's context, if you suffer prolonged periods of stress, above-average levels of cortisol will remain in your bloodstream. This means your appetite will remain high with the result that **you will constantly feel hungry**. You then eat to satisfy your hunger. As a consequence your insulin level will rise, causing it to do what it does best – store energy. Insulin stuffs more fat into your fat cells. **You put on weight**.

The hunger you experience from too much cortisol has a particular effect. It pressures you into craving foods that deliver lots of instant energy. So you crave sugar. Calorie-dense, fatty, sugary snacks from vending machines have a particular appeal. They're the ones that do you the most harm.

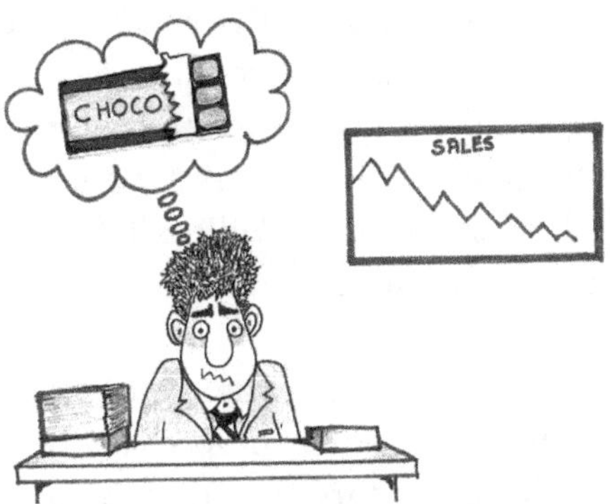

If that wasn't bad enough, prolonged exposure to high levels of cortisol also reduces the secretion of certain anabolic hormones. The effect of this is that your body loses muscle and your metabolic rate is reduced – that's the rate your body breaks down and processes energy.

Stress and fat

When you suffer from prolonged periods of stress, levels of cortisol rise, **but levels of insulin rise too.** This sends a powerful message to your fat cells to store all the energy they can and to hold onto your fat stores. In our evolutionary past, this was just in case there was another 'threat' – another sabre-toothed tiger round the corner. The effect of this is to reduce your body's ability to call on its fat stores to use as energy. Your energy storage parking attendant becomes obstinate and unhelpful and you retain fat that you need to burn.

When the cause of you being overweight or obese is down to stress, it becomes very difficult to lose fat if you remain stressed. Identifying the causes of stress, and reducing stress has to be a priority.

There is an even more important reason why reducing stress is vital, in fact it's *the* most important reason why you have to address this problem.

The fat that stress causes is different from the subcutaneous fat you have immediately under your skin which covers most of your body. Fat caused by stress is called **visceral or toxic fat**. It's the fat on your belly. It's also the fat that builds up round your internal organs. This fat is particularly dangerous. It's called toxic for a very good reason. Why? Because it drives inflammation.

What does that mean? Toxic fat is dangerous because it secretes a pro-inflammatory chemical which exacerbates the early symptoms of disease. In other words it puts you in increased danger of type 2 diabetes, of cardiovascular disease or of getting cancer. And if you don't get rid of your toxic fat, it can reduce your life by up to fifteen years. As you can see, if you're overweight or obese a lot of very nasty things can happen to you.

Now, here is *some* good news and some not so good news about fat. The good news is that it's the toxic or visceral fat is the first to go when you start to lose weight, particularly when you take regular exercise, particularly aerobic exercise. The not so good news is that your subcutaneous fat which covers most of your body is more difficult to lose. Your body tries to hang on to this **because it's this fat that makes leptin.**

Prolonged periods of stress makes you put on fat, dangerous toxic fat. Identifying the causes of stress and finding ways of coping with them is vital if you want to lose weight, and reduce the chances of contracting a life-threatening disease.

The easiest way to reduce stress and get your cortisol level down is … aerobic exercise!

Processed Food – Dark Secrets

Too many processed food products are high in SUGAR, and contain very little fibre. As you've seen, too much sugar and too little fibre in your diet are two of the prime causes of your evolutionary mismatch and the malfunction of your biochemical processes.

There are three other ingredients which, when eaten in quantity, contribute to the problem. They are **salt, fat and caffeine.**

The truth about salt

You need salt and your body is very good at extracting the salt it needs from the food you eat. Why do you need salt? You need it to regulate your fluid balance and for cardiovascular function. It also helps to make your muscles and nerves work.

The problem with the modern diet is that it contains a lot of salt. Why? Because food companies add it to processed foods as a preservative to prolong shelf life. It's also added to give food more taste.

Salt is a very effective way of enhancing flavour and attracting your approval. There's method in the madness of food manufacturers because the more salt you eat, the more you want. By adding salt it pushes your preferences, nudges your decision making towards products that have a higher salt content. If you get used to a higher level of salt in your food, it becomes the standard you expect and prefer. You're more likely to buy products that meet the standard you've become used to.

What happens when you eat too much salt?

Eating too much salt compromises kidney function.

The job of your kidneys is to filter water from your blood and send any excess to your bladder. The effect of eating too much salt is that it raises the sodium content in your blood. This disrupts your kidneys' delicate filtering process to such an extent that it reduces their ability to remove water. Instead, the water that would be have been cleared from your system by your kidneys gets stored.

The effect of storing water is that it **raises your blood pressure**. This puts strain on your arteries, your heart and your brain, which can lead to heart attack and stroke.

Eating too much salt is not only dangerous to your general health, it will cause you to put on weight. However, the weight won't come from added body fat, but from water retention. Get your salt intake right and the weight created by water retention will disappear.

Oh, there's more …

Too much salt makes you thirsty. But if you quench your thirst with a sugary or sweetened drink, it *will* lead to an increase in body fat. Potato chips followed by a Pepsi for instance. A snack high in salt and saturated fat followed by a drink full of sugar / sweeteners is the perfect storm! And guess what? Pepsi have a company that makes potato chips!

*The **RDA** (Recommended Daily Allowance) of salt is **6 grams**.*

Good fat, bad fat

There are two types of fat you should to be aware of: saturated fat and unsaturated fat. As a simple guide, **saturated fat = bad fat** and **unsaturated fat = good fat.**

Fat is not bad for you, but too much fat is, particularly saturated fat. Too much fat = too much energy, and what's surplus to your energy requirements gets stored – which leads to weight gain.

For the last forty years the food industry has been marketing 'low fat' processed foods because the perceived wisdom was that saturated fat was the cause of weight gain, obesity and associated diseases. Whilst too much fat in your diet can cause these problems, it is by no means the sole cause.

Remember, view anything labelled 'low fat' with suspicion. Don't forget the food manufacturers' sleight of hand, reducing fat in so-called 'low fat' products and replacing it with sugar. A taste enhancer it might be, but it comes at a cost to you. Remember too that 50% of sugar is fructose, and almost all fructose is metabolised as … **FAT**. 'Low fat' can actually mean 'high fat'.

By far the most toxic use of fat in food production is when it is mixed with sugar in significant quantities.

This produces a combination that is difficult to resist. The fat enhances the taste and the sugar pushes all the buttons of your reward mechanism. And some also contain high levels of salt to prompt your preferences.

You crave more. A food manufacturer's dream, a perfect alchemy, and your worst nightmare.

Examples? Cheeseburgers and fries, vanilla shakes, Danish pastries, cakes, donuts, cookies, ice cream …there's a long, long list.

Caffeine

Ask any food manufacturer why they include caffeine in their soft drinks and you'll be told that it's used to enhance flavour. It might well do, but what it really does is to give the drink extra 'edge', or to put it bluntly, it gets you 'on the hook' because caffeine is addictive, and it's also a stimulant.

You can very easily build up a dependence on caffeine. It has just the same dependence characteristics as heroin or cocaine. The more you have the more you want, and you experience withdrawal symptoms when you try to reduce your caffeine intake. It's also a diuretic – it dehydrates you. This just what you don't need if you have raised blood pressure, a condition you are very likely to have if you are overweight or obese.

When you combine the rewarding properties of sugar, (or sweeteners) and caffeine together you have a highly potent combination. Little wonder why we drink so many sugar / sweetener-laced, caffeine enhanced so-called 'sports drinks'. These make an unhelpful contribution to the evolutionary mismatch and to the malfunction of your biochemical processes.

Can food be addictive?

The reality is that we have become addicted to food, at least to processed food and to sugary, caffeinated drinks. Why? Because food manufacturers have deliberately given them addictive qualities so that we consume more, and consequently we buy more.

Excessive amounts of addictive sugar, combinations of sugar and fat that are irresistibly rewarding, salt that pressures our preferences, and caffeine that gets you on the hook…food manufacturers know how to press the right buttons. Your greed for their addictive processed products has been deliberately stimulated to satisfy their greed for profits. Unbeknown to you, the effect of their processed concoctions has put them in control – of your weight, and your health – because your biochemistry, your ability to control what and how much you eat, has been hijacked.

You are being used …for profit.

You suffer the consequences.

The quality and make-up of the processed foods you eat is what is causing you to have a weight problem, because your body cannot process them.

It doesn't have to be this way. With your determination and with the help of the Slim Habit you can take back control of your weight and your health.

It's All About Balance ...

Your body is always trying to keep things in balance, to keep everything as constant as possible. It's your hypothalamus – remember the part it plays in managing your energy balance – that's constantly interacting and adjusting to changes in order to maintain the right degree of constancy. This 'balancing act' is called homeostasis.

It's also important to keep the type of nutrients you eat in balance too. You should eat protein, fat and carbohydrate in roughly these proportions:

Protein 20%; Fat 30%; Carbohydrate 50%

Your body requires all three of these macronutrients to function properly.

Protein

Proteins are the building blocks of life. They are essential nutrients made up of amino acids which your body needs to function properly. Your tissues and organs cannot exist without proteins. Your cells contain thousands of proteins. Like tiny machines, they make your cells work. Your muscles, skin and bone contain protein. They also work as neurotransmitters and carry oxygen in your blood.

You need protein in your diet so that your body can grow. Your body also needs protein to help repair cells and make new ones. It's also a source of energy. When protein enters your digestive system it gets broken down into amino acids. Your body needs enough of these to maintain you in good health. What is enough? About 20% of your daily food intake should be protein.

There are two types of protein, animal protein and plant-sourced protein. Examples of animal protein are meats, milk, fish and eggs. Plant sources of proteins are whole grains, pulses, beans, soy and nuts.

Fat

You need fat. Dietary fat is a source of energy. It also helps your body to store and absorb fat soluble vitamins A, D, E and K. They're important because they help to regulate your blood pressure and heart rate. Dietary fats are also essential for your growth and development and for cell function.

Fat is made up of fatty acids. It's the type and the amount of fatty acids in the foods you eat that's important because of the effect they can have on your health – and your weight. You need to pay attention to **the total amount of fat you eat – and the type of fat you eat.**

There are two types of fat, saturated fat and unsaturated fat. A normal diet will contain both, but you should be aware that you need to limit the amount of saturated fat you eat because:

Saturated fat is bad fat. It's found in meat products such as sausages, a lot of processed foods, full-fat dairy products such as hard cheese, butter and cream; lard, pastry, cakes, cookies and palm oil. Why is it bad for you? Because too much saturated fat in your diet raises total blood cholesterol levels, and your LDL cholesterol (bad cholesterol) level in particular. This can lead to heart attack, stroke and type 2 diabetes.

Unsaturated fat is good fat. There are three types, monounsaturated, polyunsaturated and Omega 3 fatty acids. *Monounsaturated and polyunsaturated* fat is normally liquid at room temperature and is mainly found in plant oils such as olive and sunflower oil.

Monounsaturated fat stimulates your liver metabolism. It has a beneficial effect on your blood cholesterol levels, which can reduce your risk of heart attack or stroke. It can also benefit your insulin levels and blood sugar control and is found in oils such as olive and canola.

Polyunsaturated fat can also improve your blood cholesterol levels and is found in plant-based foods and oils.

Omega 3 fatty acids are especially good for your heart. They help to reduce the risk of you developing coronary artery disease and help to lower your blood pressure level.

Omega 3 fatty acids are found in oily fish such as mackerel and in sardines, salmon, tuna and trout. They're also found in plant sources such as flaxseed and soya bean oils, and in nuts and seeds.

Fat is a brilliant source of energy and an essential part of your diet, but it's important that you eat the right sort of fat and keep within your recommended daily allowance.

Your fat **RDA** *(Recommended Daily Allowance) is:* ***Total fats: 70 grams; Saturated fat: 20 grams***.

Carbohydrate

Like protein and fat, carbohydrate is a macronutrient. Carbohydrate provides your body, your muscles, brain and central nervous system, with the energy they need to function properly. It's your main fuel source.

There are three types of carbohydrate:
- Sugar
- Starch
- Fibre

Sugar is what is called a simple carbohydrate. Starch and fibre are both complex carbohydrates. The difference between simple and complex carbohydrates? The chemical structure is different, but in straightforward terms, you absorb simple carbohydrates more quickly. They deliver more immediate energy.

Simple carbohydrates include natural sugars found in fruit, vegetables and some milk products. And then there's the sugar added to processed food and drinks by food manufacturers, too often in unhealthy quantities.

Starch and fibre are complex carbohydrates. Starch takes much longer to be absorbed. Examples of starch are food made from grains such a bread and pasta, peas, beans, potatoes, brown rice and lentils.

All sugar and starches are broken down into simple sugars during digestion and are then absorbed into your bloodstream and known as blood sugar or blood glucose. Any excess blood glucose which you don't require for your immediate energy needs is stored in your liver, muscles and other cells, or is converted into fat.

Fibre (and there are two types) is not absorbed, but as you have seen before, soluble fibre helps prevent nutrients being absorbed too quickly, and insoluble fibre helps food progress through your gut.

Fibre should be included with your three macronutrients. A minimum of **30 grams** per day.

Essential Facts

Putting the record straight – facts you need to know

Fads, fables and fallacies abound in the world of health and weight loss. These essential facts will help to you decide between fact and fiction and give you the knowledge you need to make informed decisions.

Diets

The truth about diets? Do you lose weight when you go on a diet? Yes you do. However, in all but a tiny number of cases the weight you lose will return, usually with interest. The statement that diets make you fat isn't quite as crazy as it sounds. Remember, the diet industry makes its billions…**because diets don't work**. When one fails, you try another, and so it continues.

What happens when you go on a diet is that your body reacts by doing what it thinks is in your best interests. **It protects your fat stores.**

When you diet you reduce your food intake and, as a result, your fat cells lose fat. This causes your energy storage level to drop below normal. Your body's reaction is to produce less leptin which sends out the signal that your energy levels are low. This prompts the release of the hunger hormone, ghrelin. Guess what? You feel hungry. All you want to do is eat. **This is why dieting is difficult, and why drastic, restrictive dieting can never be a long-term weight loss solution.**

About losing weight – making change

There is no such thing as a 'quick fix' when it comes to losing weight. The quicker you lose it, the faster it will return. Successful and lasting weight loss is a gradual process, and comes from making change, learning new habits …Slim Habits.

Yes, weight gain is about eating too much, but it's more than that. It's about getting in sync with your evolutionary present. It's about what you eat and the effect the type of food you eat has on your hormones, your biochemistry. When you become overweight or obese it's your biochemistry that drives your behaviour, not you. When this happens weight gain is inevitable, and weight loss is almost impossible.

Your environment and your lifestyle also play a significant part in determining your weight and your general health. Understanding the effects they have is crucial to a positive long-term outcome. Facing up to uncomfortable truths is not easy. If you have the will to make change, the Slim Habit will help you achieve your goals.

Be careful where you put your trust – know your enemy

Surely all food is good for you? If it tastes good, stops you from feeling hungry and gives you energy, isn't that okay? Well, it might well have been okay in your evolutionary past, but today the story is a very different one.

Never before have we had such a variety of foods available to us. The supermarket shelves are groaning under the weight of beautifully packaged, tempting foods. But are they all they seem? Should we trust the branded foods we know so well?

Perhaps the question should be asked in a different way. Should we trust a lightly regulated, huge and highly profitable food industry, which uses its corporate power to influence governments to avoid regulation, to produce food that does us no harm? The clue is in the question. Where there is the opportunity for huge profits, and where those in power allow corporations to influence decisions to favour their best interests rather than for the common good, the answer has to be an emphatic 'NO'!

This is such a pity because the food industry has been hugely innovative, delivering some really fantastic, great-value products. However, some of the food that food companies produce have had a devastating effect on our bodies, our hormones, our health and our quality of life.

The amount of **SUGAR**, salt, saturated fat, the lack of essential fibre and the addition of weird and wonderful additives included by food companies' culinary alchemists, has produced processed foods that come close to being classed as toxic, when they're consumed in quantity – which so many of them are. Particularly shocking are the high levels of sugar in processed foods and drinks. No surprise that the rise in sugar consumption has gone hand-in-hand with the rise in obesity over the last thirty years.

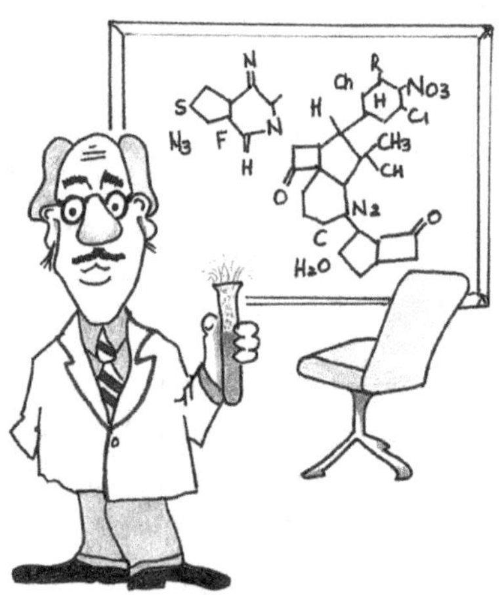

Chicken pie!

When it comes to food, you need to have trust in your own judgement. Good judgement comes from knowledge. You have to build up your knowledge about food, about how it affects you, about understanding why there is an evolutionary mismatch, and by gathering intelligence about processed food so that you will never be taken in by misleading claims and disingenuous marketing.

Water and weight loss

To work properly your body needs the fluids you drink and the water it extracts from the food you eat. Your digestive system, brain function, the biochemical reactions that go on throughout your body, the lubrication of your joints, the detoxification of your system and the regulation of your body temperature, all need water.

When you don't drink enough water you become dehydrated. The situation can be made worse if your diet contains too much salt or if you drink a lot of caffeinated drinks or your alcohol consumption is high. **Dehydration leads to water retention**. This happens when your body tries to defend your interests by retaining as much water as it can in order to keep everything working. The result? **You become bloated and you put on weight.** If you're overweight or obese, some of your extra weight will almost certainly be caused by water retention.

How much water should you drink?

How much water should you drink to avoid becoming dehydrated and to keep everything working efficiently? During a normal day you'll lose over 2 litres (3 ½ pints) of water through normal bodily functions – you lose a pint of water simply by exhaling. Some of this will be replaced by what your body extracts from the food you eat, but unless you replace what you lose – and then some – you'll become dehydrated. To avoid this happening, the simple rule is to keep your salt intake to no more than 6 grams a day, avoid caffeinated sodas, drink alcohol in moderation, and **drink at least 7–8 medium glasses** (a medium-sized glass = 8 fluid ounces / 200 ml) of water every day. The good news is that by simply following this rule you can get rid of bloating *and* lose the weight that comes with it.

The best thing to do is to start the day with a couple of glasses of water, and then spread the time you drink water throughout the day. If you drink a glass of water 30 minutes *before* you have a meal, it will help to reduce your appetite – and your calorie intake – maybe by up to 80 calories a day. That's over 8 pounds / 4 kilos in a year just by drinking the right amount of water. Do other drinks like tea and coffee count towards your overall fluid intake? Yes, they do, but it's best if you drink water in addition to any cups of tea or coffee you may have.

Be aware that the signal that you are hungry and the signal that you are thirsty are very similar and are often confused.

It's very easy to answer a thirst signal with food. The best thing to do is to always answer what you think might be a hunger signal with a glass of water. If it's a thirst signal it'll satisfy your thirst, if it really is a hunger signal it'll have reduced your appetite.

Can lack of sleep make you fat?

On average we sleep nearly two hours less than we did fifty years ago. Why? Probably because we stay up late watching television or we're glued to an iPad or laptop late into the evening. Too often we snack or eat calorie-dense, sugary, processed food and drink alcohol too close to bedtime. This raises your blood sugar level *and* makes sleep difficult. The result is that we don't get enough sleep – and what sleep we do get is unsatisfactory. We become sleep deprived, and that's not good.

When you don't get enough sleep – and it's wise to try and get as near to 7 ½ hours' sleep every night as you can – next day you'll probably find it difficult to concentrate, and you may struggle to solve simple problems. You'll be less alert, have memory lapses and you may find it difficult to reason effectively. Constant sleep deprivation can also lead to depression and to more serious diseases such as heart attack, stroke and type 2 diabetes.

Yes, it's true, lack of sleep makes you fat. Why? Because your body interprets lack of sleep as an energy deficiency. When you wake, your hunger hormone ghrelin is high and your energy storage hormone leptin is low.

At breakfast you are stimulated to put things right as quickly as possible. You crave something which will raise your blood sugar level quickly. The quickest way to do that? A slug of something sugary. This is the quickest way to get your blood sugar up and reduce your ghrelin and leptin levels. So when you appear at the breakfast table you gulp down a glass of deliciously sweet fruit juice and tuck into a heaped bowl of sugary cereal. Your blood sugar level shoots up. You feel better and your hunger pangs disappear.

However, within an hour or so of your breakfast the inevitable happens, as it always does after a sugar rush. Your blood sugar levels plummet, and soon you're on the hunt for something sweet again. More often than not this leads to a day punctuated by frequent sugary snacks. **You put on weight** as a result.

What to do …

Here are some simple rules that will help you to get a good night's sleep and stop you putting on weight:

- Try and leave a gap of **four hours** between eating your evening meal and going to sleep. If this isn't possible, eat a light meal in the evening and avoid eating anything sweet. Don't snack after your evening meal.

- If you drink more than a glass of wine or a small glass of beer in the evening, you'll fall asleep quickly, but it'll be a shallow, fragmented sleep and you'll wake up feeling tired.

- Coffee in the evening? The caffeine in coffee is a stimulant so it's best to **avoid coffee** if you want to have a good sleep. Some people don't find this a problem, but most do.

- Don't look at a light-emitting screen like an iPad or a phone, at least **one hour** before you go to bed. Why? Because it'll affect your sleep-promoting hormone melatonin. **It may reduce it by up to 50%.** You'll find it difficult to get to sleep, and it may affect the quality of your sleep for the rest of the night.

Alcohol – the 'must know' facts

Did you realise that your body sees alcohol as a poison? It doesn't like it. Not only because it believes that it'll do you harm, but **because it can't store its calories.** So when you drink alcohol, your body's first reaction is to break it down and get rid of it as quickly as possible. It immediately stops metabolising anything else, and prioritises metabolising the alcohol.

Your stomach breaks down about 10% of the alcohol, another 10% is metabolised by your brain, which is why you feel intoxicated. **The remaining 80%, like fructose, is metabolised by your liver.**

Try as it might to get alcohol out of your system quickly, **it takes your liver an hour to metabolise one alcoholic drink**. When you drink a lot of alcohol, your system becomes saturated. Alcohol accumulates in your blood until it can be metabolised by your liver, which is why the effect of drinking alcohol can last for a long time.

Drinking alcohol may be pleasurable, but you are **drinking calories**, lots of them. A 250ml glass of wine contains 280 calories, the equivalent of eating a bar of chocolate. A pint of lager contains 180 calories. Drink five pints of lager every week and you will drink 45,000 extra calories in a year. The sums are easy to do.

The problem with alcohol is that it's metabolised in the same way as fructose – as fat. (Hardly surprising, because alcohol is simply fermented sugar). Your liver converts alcohol into aldehydes, some of which is converted into glucose. The remainder forms free fatty acids and then triglycerides which are then shunted into your fat cells. The really bad news is that the fat made by alcohol is the toxic, visceral, pro-inflammatory variety that surrounds your major internal organs and manifests itself externally as – **belly fat.**

Alcohol? It makes you fat!

Drinking calories – the road to ruin?

In your evolutionary past your ancestors ate their calories. They didn't drink them.

Today, drinking calories is what we like to do. From sugar-laden carbonated sodas to fruit juices and smoothies, we can't seem to get enough of them. So much so that **30% of the SUGAR we consume comes not from what we eat, but from what we drink.**

Just one 12 oz (350 ml) can of Classic **Coke contains 39 grams of sugar, that's 10 teaspoons** – which is more than your recommended daily allowance!

(A Diet Coke contains sweeteners that may reduce your sugar intake, but will have a negative impact on your ability to lose weight, and may even cause you to put on weight.)

*The RDA (Recommended Daily Allowance) of sugar is **25 grams**. You may find it useful to remember that **4 grams of sugar = 1 teaspoon**.*

But what about orange juice, surely that's good for you? Any juice, whether it's labelled as 'not from concentrate' or not, is not what it seems. The process of juicing removes all the fibre and what you are left with is a tasty liquid full of … **SUGAR. A 17oz (500 ml) bottle of Pret orange juice contains 51 grams of sugar, over 12 teaspoons, more than a can of Coke!**

Smoothies? Smoothies are just blitzed fruit, but the process of blitzing or juicing, tears the insoluble fibre in the fruit to shreds. The soluble fibre that's left can't do the job you need it to do of forming a barrier in your gut to slow down the process of absorption. So when you savour a smoothie your liver receives an avalanche of fructose, and your pancreas responds by producing lots of insulin to deal with the avalanche. The more insulin you produce, the more fat gets stored.

An 8.5 oz (250 ml) Innocent pomegranates, blueberry and acai smoothie contains 34 grams of sugar, 8.5 teaspoons. A 500ml cup of MacDonald's mango and pineapple smoothie contains 52 grams of sugar, 13 teaspoons.

Don't forget sugar or sucrose, is made up of half glucose and half fructose and nearly all fructose is metabolised by your liver – **as fat**.

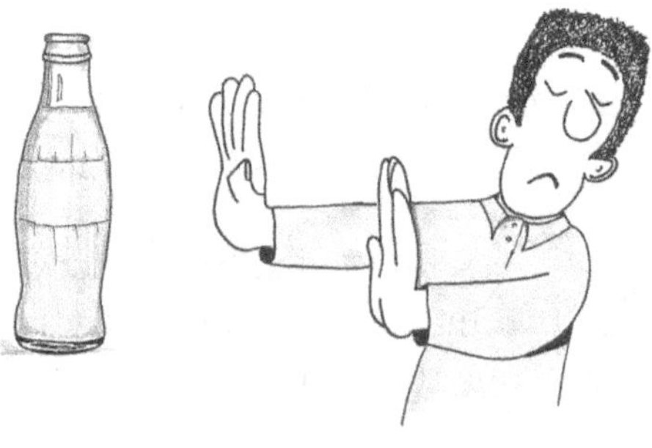

Drinking calories makes you fat!

If you're thirsty, drink water. If you like fruit, eat it, don't drink it. That way you'll eat the right amount of fibre and the fructose in the fruit will be absorbed and metabolised as it should be.

Are you still hungry? How not to over eat

Have you ever wondered why you still feel hungry having eaten a good lunch? Or maybe wondered why your body doesn't tell you when to stop eating? Actually, your body *will* tell you when you've had enough and you're full – if you let it!

As food passes through your small intestine it releases a hormone called peptide YY, or PYY. This signals to your hypothalamus that you're full. It's your satiety signal. The problem is that your small intestine is 22 feet long. The food has to travel a long way before the full signal is generated.

In your evolutionary past ...

The food your ancestors ate contained lots of fibre so it would pass through the gut quickly. It was also probably quite tough and took time to eat. Today, processed food is easy to eat. It takes no time at all to eat a meal, and as it contains very little fibre it passes through your gut slowly. It takes a long time for the PYY signal to be activated, which is why you don't feel full, and you keep eating. This is another example of being out of sync, another symptom of your evolutionary mismatch.

If it takes about 20 minutes from the time you start eating for PYY to be activated, the best way to get over this problem is to eat slowly. Take time to chew your food, avoid processed foods and eat food that contains lots of fibre – fruit and vegetables – and let your body speak to you!

To snack or not to snack, that is the question

Forty years ago there was very little snacking. Of course people ate between meals, but not as a rule. Food was eaten at meal times and children were told off if they had something to eat between meals that "spoiled their appetite". There were only a limited number of snacks you could buy, until …until food companies realised they were missing a trick.

One of the very first advertisements for snacks claimed, "The sweet you can eat between meals without spoiling your appetite". This was the Milky Bar advertisement which successfully lured children and indulgent parents into accepting the snacking habit.

Since then, food companies have been so successful in producing a vast range of tasty, sugary snacks, that snacking has become a national pastime. **A quarter of our daily calorie intake now comes from snacks** and nearly 50% of that intake is from calories we drink, from sugary beverages like sodas, fruit juices, smoothies and coffee concoctions.

To snack or not to snack? If you eat three nutritious, balanced meals a day, and keep to your recommended daily allowances, you shouldn't need to snack. If you do have a snack it should be a healthy one, a piece of fruit, not a chocolate bar. If you feel thirsty, drink water not a sugary drink. Remember that the hunger signal is easily confused with the thirst signal. Don't grab a snack, answer the signal with a glass of water. **Treat snacks as an occasional treat, not something that is a part of your regular diet.**

Give your body a break, not a snack!

The importance of eating breakfast

Breakfast is the most important meal of the day. Have a good breakfast and you will set yourself up for the day. You'll feel more energetic, you'll perform better, and you won't feel the need to snack.

Skipping breakfast sets you off on the wrong foot. Skip it, and you won't have suppressed your hunger hormone ghrelin. It won't be long before you feel really hungry and your blood sugar hits rock bottom. You start to crave a sugary snack. Before you know it you're off to the vending machine.

And your day won't get any better. It's been shown that if you don't have a good breakfast, you'll have food on your mind all day. Why? Because your ghrelin level remains high. As a result you'll feel hungry throughout the day. You'll eat too many calories at lunch, eat more snacks in the afternoon, and cap the day off with a large meal before you go to bed. All this will make you put on weight … and all because you skipped breakfast.

Some people say that they don't want to eat breakfast because they don't feel hungry. The cause? Probably the most common cause is eating a large meal too late in the evening, having a late snack or drinking alcohol before you turn in. Shovelling energy into your body just at the time when it needs it least is not a good idea. If you do, most of the energy will be stored as fat because you don't need it, and that's why you won't feel hungry in the morning.

Not getting up early enough to give yourself enough time to eat breakfast or being in a rush in the morning can also get you into the habit of not eating breakfast. Adjust your routine to make sure you have time for breakfast.

What's a good breakfast? **One which contains about a quarter of your daily calories.** Why? Because you need to kick start your body's energy-burning process and eat enough food to keep your hunger hormone ghrelin at bay.

What to eat for breakfast?

It takes energy to burn food – approximately 200 calories a day – and it takes twice the amount of energy to burn protein as it does carbohydrate. This has the effect of reducing your appetite. Including protein in your breakfast makes sense – "going to work on an egg" is a very good idea.

As well as protein, a non-sugary cereal to will give you the minerals and vitamins you need, and a piece of fresh fruit will add essential fibre to your breakfast. Remember not to add sugar to your cereal, your coffee or tea, and avoid sugar-loaded fruit juice and smoothies.

Control your hunger pangs – eat a good breakfast!

When to eat

The old saying 'breakfast like a king, lunch like a prince and dine like a pauper' is actually very sensible advice. A really good breakfast is the best way to start the day. Lunch should be sufficient so that you don't feel the need to snack during the afternoon. Your evening meal should be light and eaten as early as is practicable.

When you eat can be dictated by the requirements of your daily life, but there are serious health benefits to be had if you can reduce the time between meals and by doing so **lengthen the time when you are not eating** i.e. the time between your evening meal and breakfast. Why? Because what you are doing in effect is to have a mini fast. Providing you don't snack or drink alcohol after your evening meal this is the time when your body is free from processing food and when it can turn its attention to some timely repairs and maintenance. It will also help to **reduce your body fat and lower your blood sugar and cholesterol levels.**

Recommended Daily Allowances

When it comes to losing weight or maintaining your weight, your focus needs to be on keeping within your recommended daily allowances. **Keeping within your RDA for total fat, saturated fat, sugar and salt, and eating the right amount of fibre,** is the best way of keeping a check on what you're eating, and the best way to help you to make better food choices.

Eating an excessive number of calories is obviously not good, but it's when you exceed the recommended daily allowances for total fat, saturated fat, sugar and salt, that your problems start.

It's not difficult to build up your knowledge about the quantities of nutrients in the food you eat. Becoming aware of what they are is the first step.

Here are the Recommended Daily Allowances, RDAs, for the nutrients total fat, saturated fat, sugar, salt and for fibre

Nutrient	Total
Total Fat	70 grams
Saturated Fat	20 grams
Sugar	25 grams*
Salt	6 grams
Fibre	30 grams

*This is the RDA for 'free sugar' which is sugar added by a food manufacturer and any sugars present in honey, syrups and fruit juices. You don't need to worry about the naturally occurring sugar in milk (maltose) or in whole fruit and vegetables.

The World Health Organisation recommends that your RDA for sugar should be 25 grams, 6¼ teaspoons. 25 grams is the level recommended by the Slim Habit. (RDA, Recommended Daily Allowance is the same as RI, which is an abbreviation for Reference Intake)

Fibre

30 grams is the daily **minimum** number of grams of fibre you should eat. The more fibre you eat the better. Remember your ancestors consumed up to 100 grams.

Understanding Food Labels

Food labels have all the information you need to help you stay within your RDA (Recommended Daily Allowance) of sugar, salt, total fat, saturated fat and fibre.

It takes a little bit of practice to interpret some of these labels, but it's easy once you get used to it. You'll soon be able to glance at a label and get the information you want. Labels vary slightly, but here's how you can make sense of them.

Typical Food Label

UK food label example

		Typical value per 100g	Per 30g serving
→	ENERGY	1604kJ 378kcal	481kJ 113kcal
→ →	FAT of which saturates	0.9g 0.2g	0.3g 0.1g
→	CARBOHYDRATES of which sugars	84g 8g	25g 2.4g
→	FIBRE	3g	0.9g
	PROTEIN	7g	2.1g
→	SALT	1.13g	0.34g

US food label example

		% Daily Value
→	**Total Fat** 8g	10
→	Saturated Fat 1g	5
	Trans Fat 0g	
	Cholesterol 0mg	0
→	**Sodium** 160mg	7
	Total Carbohydrate 37g	13
→	Dietary Fibre 4g	14
	Total Sugars 12g	
→	Includes 10g Added Sugars	20
	Protein 3g	

Category 'ENERGY'

The first category on every label is the ENERGY value. On the UK label this is expressed in kcal, i.e. calories. With the Slim Habit you won't be counting calories, (except on Low Calorie Days) but the kcal (calorie) value gives you, at a glance, a very good indication of whether or not it's a high-calorie product or not. For example, if you take 2000 calories as a daily base-line calorie intake for an average adult, from the example above, a 30g serving would be 113 kcal (calories), which is 6% of base line calorie intake, so not high.

Category 'FAT'

This is number of grams of **total fat**, that contains both saturated fat (bad fat) and unsaturated fat (good fat) – RDA 70 grams.

You are interested in the total fat content because this figure tells you if the product is high in fat or not.

'**Of which sarurates**': is the number of grams of **saturated** fat – bad fat – RDA 20 grams.

*This is a **crucial figure**, and will tell you how much bad fat the product contains.*

Category 'CARBOHYDRATES'

You are interested in the **'of which sugars'** figure. Look for the number of grams of sugar in the product – RDA 25 grams

Category 'SALT'

The total quantity of salt expressed in grams – RDA 6 grams.

Salt is 40% sodium and 60% chloride. It's the sodium that's the 'bad part', so be careful when you see a label that lists sodium rather than salt. High sodium products need to be avoided. You have to multiply the amount of sodium by 2.5 to get the amount of salt. So your RDA of 6 grams is equal to 2.4 grams of sodium.

Category 'FIBRE'

The number of grams of fibre. Unlike the other nutrition types above, the higher the figure the better – RDA >30 grams.

Guidelines – how to make a quick judgement

This table shows guideline amounts for you to be able to judge whether a nutrient is high or low. If you can memorise these you might find it helpful. At a glance you will be able to make a judgement about whether you should buy the product or not.

Nutrient	High (per 100g)	Low (per 100g)	RDA
Total Fat	>17.5g	<5g	70g
Saturated Fat	>5g	<1.5g	20g
Sugar	>22.5g	<5g	25g
Salt	>1.5g	<0.3	6g
Sodium (mg)	>620mg	<125mg	2479mg

Portions, servings and slices

Some labels give nutrient amounts by portion size. This can be helpful, but be careful because the manufacturer's idea of a portion size may be deliberately small and different to yours.

Traffic light labelling

Some supermarkets use this quick referencing system. Normally it refers to the content of Fat (total fat) Saturates (saturated fat) Sugars and Salt in a product. **Green is low, amber is medium and red is high**. There is no traffic light for fibre. Traffic light labelling is a useful guide, but it's always best to check the proper label as well.

Consequences

Life's one long feast

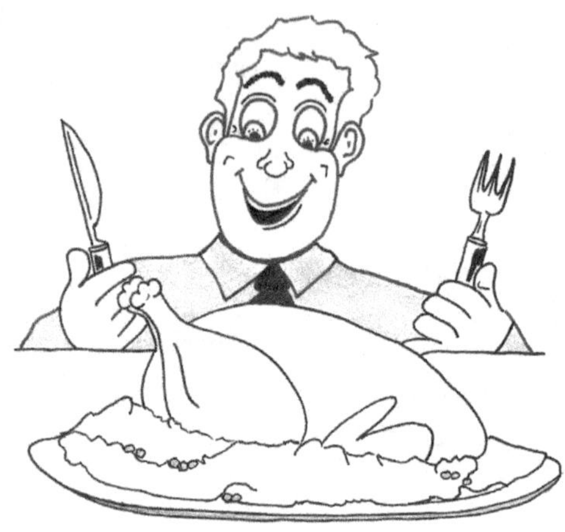

Your hunter gatherer ancestors led a very different life from yours. They experienced both periods of plenty and periods of famine. Like you, their bodies evolved over many hundreds of thousands of years, developed hugely sophisticated ways of ensuring they could survive famine as well as times when food was scarce. It had a reward system that encouraged them to eat when food was plentiful, and an energy storage system that squirreled away surplus energy into their fat cells as a reserve they could call upon when food was scarce. One thing you can be sure of is that with a life punctuated by feast and famine, they didn't have a weight problem.

Actually, lean times and periods of famine were important for their health and survival. Why? Because when there was a shortage of food and there was little or no food to process, **their bodies were programmed to carry out repairs and maintenance. Famine or lack of food, switched on a repair gene.** Faulty cells were repaired, bad cells were disposed of and new ones created, and their immune system regenerated. This process of creating more cells and regenerating the immune system increased their ability to resist infections and reduced the risk of developing diseases, including cancer.

This wasn't something that happened just because the body had nothing else to do. It had developed to become an essential part of how the body kept itself 'in tune', making sure it was working as efficiently as possible, keeping healthy and free from disease.

Your body is no different. In evolutionary terms your body is the same as your ancestors'. Nothing has changed. What has changed though, is your lifestyle and your behaviour.

Your reward system and your energy storage system work perfectly well …if they are not compromised by what you eat. And your repair gene? It still exists. But it needs to be activated to do essential repairs and maintenance. Does this happen? No! Why? Because you don't let it. There is never any famine or any time when you have very little to eat …you never give it a chance to get to work.

Constant eating, snacking or gulping down sugary drinks means there's never a sufficient gap when you are not eating for your repair gene to get to work, to do essential repairs and maintenance. Cells are not repaired or replaced as they should be, and your immune system is not regenerated. In these days of perpetual feast, the essential process of repairs and maintenance just doesn't happen. And the consequences? Weight gain and the prospect of bad health.

Get in sync!

Sign up to the logic of 'Low Calorie Days'

Perversely, **Low Calorie Days** and periods of famine were important to your ancestors. They wouldn't have known it, but these lean days of little food kept them slim. **Days when you eat very little are as**

important to you today as they were to your ancestors in your evolutionary past.

Low Calorie Days

Your body still thinks it's a hunter gatherer – and it is. It's still programmed to handle feast and famine and it still needs days when it has time off from processing food. This is your cue to help your body, and to help yourself.

What is a Low Calorie Day? They are often called **fast days**, but to some, fast implies you eat nothing at all. On Low Calorie Days you do eat, but you significantly reduce what you eat. **A diet of 550 calories is a Low Calorie Day.** The calories you eat should include a combination **of what you eat normally**, that is a mixture of protein, fat and carbohydrate.

Introducing LCDs (Low Calorie Days) into your life does two things:

1. It reconnects you to your evolutionary present, gets you back in sync, and gives your body the time it needs to switch on its repair genes and do essential repairs and maintenance.

2. It gives you a simple and effective tool with which to manage your weight.

Low Calorie Days and weight management

Low Calorie Days are a highly effective way of managing your weight and of getting – and remaining – healthy. They are a common-sense way of mobilising your body's naturally evolved systems, to work *for* you and not *against* you.

Low Calorie Days work best when you combine them with two things:

1. You eat sensibly on normal days. 'Sensibly' means keeping as near as you possible can to your Recommended Daily Allowance for sugar, salt, fat and saturated fat and fibre.

2. You take regular exercise.

The bonus of Low Calorie Days? **The weight you lose when you go on a Low Calorie Day is nearly all fat. There is almost no muscle loss**. (With most diets you will lose as much muscle as you do fat. This doesn't happen with Low Calorie Days)

Managing your Low Calorie days

You can use Low Calorie Days in a number of different ways. They will always have an positive effect on your general health and your weight. Two Low Calorie Days each week is recommended for best results.

* **Two Low Calorie Days a week** (on non-consecutive days). Not only will these deliver gradual weight loss, you'll find your cholesterol levels will improve, you'll get rid of your toxic fat, and your waistline will become smaller – and as an added bonus, you'll feel great.

* **Add another day.** You can add another day and do **three Low Calorie Days** a week (on non-consecutive days). This will produce faster results, but if you decide to do 3 LCD's it might be better to do it every other week.

* **Alternate day Low Calorie Days** This is quite hardcore and you may find this difficult to do. Obviously you will lose more weight

the more days you do, but it's unwise to overdo it. A gradual approach is more likely to produce better long-term results.

- **One Low Calorie Day a week.** Once you've reached your target weight it's a good idea to have at least one low calorie day every week to keep 'in tune', to support your general wellbeing and manage your weight.

A Low Calorie Day is always useful following a day when you've eaten more than you should. It gets you back to where you were. Yes, you can enjoy yourself and still be in control of your weight!

Be patient

When starting to do Low Calorie Days it's a good idea to take things slowly. When you first start, the thought of eating very little for a whole day can be a little daunting, but when you've done it once or twice you'll think nothing of it. If you include protein in what you eat for breakfast it will help stave off any hunger pangs and you probably won't feel as though you want anything to eat until lunchtime. Towards the end of the day you'll be surprised by how good you feel – and that you're not craving food. Remember to keep drinking water!

What about normal days?

On normal days, there is no restriction on what you eat. All you have to do is to keep as near as you can to your RDA of sugar, fibre, salt, fat and saturated fat. This still gives you a huge choice of amazing food to eat, but it will mean eating less processed food, ready meals and fast food – and an end to drinking calories from fruit juices, smoothies and sugar-laced drinks. As an added bonus you'll find that the quality of what you eat will improve.

What do you think your hunter gatherer ancestors looked like? In a word, lean. Although there would be times of feast when they would gain weight, it would have been highly unlikely if any of them were overweight. Days when they had very little to eat, low calorie days, would have kept their weight in check. Low calorie days can do the same for you too.

Getting in sync: Stop eating food that does you harm!

It's the quality of the food you eat that's the root cause of your evolutionary mismatch. You've been pushed out of the driving seat and your biochemistry is in control of what you eat and how much you eat. **But now at least you know!**

You now have the knowledge and understanding about how your body reacts to what you eat and the consequences that follow. You know what causes your evolutionary mismatch. Now you can do something about it.

Eating the right food

Diets tell you what food to eat. Their prescriptive regimes eventually turn your life into a nightmare – and put you off trying to lose weight. They are unsustainable.

If you understand what processed foods can do to you, if you're aware what causes your biochemistry to be turned on its head, you can make informed choices about what you eat and drink. The best way to do this is not to become a slave to a list of food and drink you are allowed or not allowed, but **simply keep as near as you can to the Recommended Daily Allowances for sugar, salt, fat, saturated fat and fibre.**

Common sense choices

By keeping to the Recommended Daily Allowance for sugar, salt, fat, saturated fat and fibre you will find that you will be steered towards healthier food, more common-sense choices, choices that help you to keep within the RDAs.

Time and patience

It takes time and patience at the beginning to get used to the labels and keeping score. **But the bonus is that you can choose whatever you want to buy and to eat as long as you keep within your RDAs.**

Much of what you do initially will be about finding alternatives to the products you normally buy, and then when you get home, working out how much you can eat. We all tend to buy very similar things every week so eventually shopping and meal planning will become easy. It's all about becoming aware of new choices, and there are plenty of them.

Getting in Sync – Exercise, loading the silver bullet!

Exercise is primarily about health and well-being. You won't lose weight just by taking exercise, but you *will* put on weight if you don't take exercise.

Why? Because if you don't take regular exercise your body, your systems, don't function properly. Exercise keeps you 'in tune'. When you don't take exercise your weight increases – and you put yourself in line to succumb to some very nasty diseases that could ruin, and shorten, your life.

If you want to lose weight and maintain your weight loss, exercise has to be part of what you do. Here is how exercise makes a difference:

- **Exercise, aerobic exercise, exercise that gets your heart beating faster, gets rid of toxic visceral fat**, the fat that collects around your major organs such as your heart, liver and intestines and which also manifests itself as belly fat. This toxic, pro-inflammatory fat can cause cardiovascular disease, insulin resistance leading to type 2 diabetes, and cancer. The good news is that visceral fat is the fat that goes first when you start to take regular exercise.

- **Exercise improves your metabolic state**, in other words it improves the efficiency of the chemical reactions in your body and specifically your *calorie burning efficiency*. You work better.

- **By building muscle through exercise you improve your insulin sensitivity** and your and insulin levels are lowered. Exercise also improves leptin signalling and makes your internal communication systems work properly. You start to function efficiently.

- **Exercise is the best way to reduce stress**. By managing your stress level through exercise you reduce, if not eliminate, cortisol from your system. Remember cortisol increases your appetite, particularly for sugary carbohydrates. Exercise to reduce stress and prevent weight gain.

Exercise is the best way to improve your health.

Other benefits of regular exercise? It is an anti-depressant, it improves your cognative function and you'll live longer.

Exercise shouldn't be a chore, it should be what you do. It needs to become part of your daily routine – and something you enjoy. The more you do, the more you will enjoy it, particularly when you start to experience the benefits.

See Part Four – Exercise for you

Your Evolutionary Inheritance

Your evolutionary inheritance is a gift. But, as you've seen, if you don't appreciate what it is, if you don't understand how to keep in sync with it, it will work against you.

Your amazing body has evolved over millions of years. In all those years there has been one purpose behind the evolutionary changes that have taken place – your survival. Everything about you has evolved to give you the best chance of surviving.

From now on you should have in the back of your mind that you were, and still are, a highly efficient hunter gatherer. In evolutionary terms that's where you're at. But society, our lifestyle habits and our diet have evolved at such breakneck speed that we are now faced with an evolutionary mismatch which is a serious threat to our weight, our well-being and our health. We are out of sync. If this problem is not addressed – if *you* don't address the problem – it will have far-reaching consequences. The way to avoid those consequences and have a slim, healthy life is to make change.

So here's what to do next …

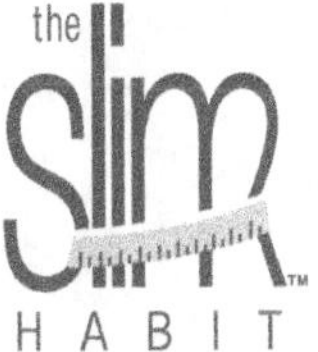

Part Two

Preparation

Knowledge is the key to making successful change. It allows you to 'own' the change process because you know what causes you to be overweight; you know about the evolutionary mismatch, of the effects of your biochemistry driving your behaviour, and how it affects your weight and your health.

In Part One 'What you need to know' you have been made aware of things that you need to change, and that hopefully you want to change.

The next stage is to for you to prepare your own Slim Habit programme. A slim, healthy life is yours for the taking.

Your Slim Habit will be based on three main areas: **Your Diet, Low Calorie Days and Exercise**. It won't be like a diet, restrictive and short-lasting. It will be simple, easy to follow and easy to do. **The new habits you learn will become part of your life, for the rest of your life**. Your Slim Habit programme will be 'owned' by you and controlled by you. You'll be able to adjust it whenever you feel the need to do so.

Your new slim, healthy life starts here, but before getting down to the detail, there's some personal preparation to do. Here are two things you'll find helpful to be aware of ...

About habits

In order to make change you're going to have to change your habits. So what is a habit? A habit is a familiar activity carried out automatically, without much thought. It's a learned response. We live our lives mostly by habit. For example, after a few months of learning to ride a bike or drive a car, we can do it 'without thinking'. It becomes automatic. It's because we've done it repeatedly that it's becomes a habit. The fact that we're able to form habits allows us a huge amount of freedom. It frees our brain to be able to concentrate on more pressing issues. It makes us more efficient.

Often we're not aware that we're learning a habit. It becomes established because we do something repeatedly. Routines, for example. It's easy to become hampered by routine. Routines develop without you being aware. Routines are how you run much of your life. They are just a collection of habits, some good, some bad. By learning new habits you can deconstruct your routines and create new ones. It's not difficult to do, it might take a bit of getting used to at first, but it's necessary – and it works.

Repetition and practice is what creates habit!

Habits can work *for* us, and *against* us. Sitting down every evening and watching TV can become a habit. Not taking exercise can become a habit. Buying the same brand of sugary drink can become a habit. Not eating breakfast can become a habit. Snacking can become a habit. Taking lunch at McDonalds can become a habit. The secret about making change is that …

If you want to change a habit you have to learn a new one!

You can't 'unlearn' a habit, but **you can learn a new one to take its place**. You've heard of habits becoming 'ingrained'. What this really means is that your brain is happy with the way things are and doesn't want to change. Because your habits have become 'what you do' it believes it's in your best interests to maintain the status quo.

The way to change this is to make your brain aware of what you want to do. You do this by focusing on what you want to achieve and then mentally rehearsing what you would do. For example, focus on making a success of your Low Calorie Day and then mentally rehearse what you're going to do. This prepares your brain for change and sets up new connections which will help you to overcome your brain's natural resistance to change. Repetition of the habit will deliver the change you want to make. A good thing to remember is that..

Change is just another word for learning!

Successful change comes not from amending or altering an existing habit, but by replacing it – by **learning a new habit**, and then practicing it until it becomes ingrained, hotwired in your brain.

How long does it take to learn a new habit? 21 days is a good rule of thumb, but the more you practice the more ingrained your new habit will become.

Your Slim Habit programme is about identifying old habits you need to change and learning new ones. It's about making long-term changes in your behaviour that will deliver weight loss and enable you to take control of your weight and your health. And here's something which will help you … visualisation.

Visualising the new you

Making change takes determination and resolve. Visualisation can be very helpful when it comes to strengthening your determination and resolve. What is visualisation? It's about creating images in your mind. In other words, using the power of your imagination to help you to focus on what you want to achieve. Just picture in your mind's eye for a moment, how you would like to look. Well, there's absolutely no reason why that *can't* be you! This imagining, rehearsing of what you want the outcome to be can be very powerful.

It has the effect of pre-activating your brain to expect something new. It makes your goals much easier to achieve. Why? Because your brain is not playing catch-up, or fighting to make sense of a new situation. You're pre-warning it and preparing it to be ready to support you.

All you have to do is to take a few quiet moments to visualise what you intend to do and reflect on what you want the ultimate outcome to be. Keep that image in your mind.

You'll find your first Low Calorie Day much less of a challenge if you visualise what you plan to do and the positive outcome it and subsequent days will have on your weight and your health. Your brain will understand what is happening when you change your eating habits, you'll be mentally prepared, and you'll find it much easier to do.

Decision time – choose a date

You need time to prepare before you start your Slim Habit. How long you take before you start is entirely up to you, but it might be sensible to **have an idea of when you want to start and set a date** so that you can focus your mind on your preparation. Probably best if you read what you have to prepare first, then decide. Here's what you need to do to prepare.

Your diet

Preparation – food awareness

There's no restriction on what you eat or drink on your Slim Habit programme (except on Low Calorie Days), **BUT** the one thing you have to do is to try to keep as near as you can to your Recommended Daily Allowance for total fat, saturated fat, sugar, fibre and salt. This will mean that your meal choices will have to change or be amended.

First, it's a good idea to make yourself aware of the total fat, saturated fat, sugar, fibre and salt that's in what you are **currently eating and drinking**. The best way to do this is to pull out all the food you have from your store cupboards, your fridge and your freezer and have a good look at what you've got. Seeing what your current diet looks like when it's laid out in front of you will be revealing, but hopefully informative too. It'll also give you the opportunity to get used to reading food labels.

> ***Tip:*** *Why not make a list? On the left hand side write down the item and then make five columns headed: total fat, saturated fat, sugar, fibre, salt. Enter the number of grams per 100 grams in the appropriate column. Apart from seeing the quantities of sugar, salt etc., in the food you've been eating, you'll find this list useful when you have to make decisions about what to buy when you go shopping.*

Let's start with drinks.

Drinks

Open up your store cupboards, the fridge, wherever you keep your stash of sugary drinks. Dig out all the bottles of soda, cans of Coke, cartons of fruit juice and smoothies.

Now take a good look at the labels and the amount of sugar they contain. Have in mind that your RDA (Recommended Daily Allowance) of sugar is 25 grams. Some drinks, particularly so-called diet drinks will contain sweeteners. Drinks containing sweeteners consumed in quantity will, as you have seen, very much work against your efforts to lose weight.

Separate 'good' drinks and say goodbye to the bad ones. Yes, drinks where sugar has been substituted by sweeteners are in the bad category.

Drink them if you must or give them away, but get rid of them before your start date.

And what about alcohol? Well, bear in mind that alcohol makes you fat. If you've got the odd few cans of beer or a bottle of wine or two, put them in an out-of-the-way cupboard away from temptation. An occasional drink is not going to be ruled out forever, but it's best do without alcohol until you feel you've have made real progress with your Slim Habit. Thereafter alcohol in moderation is fine.

Eat your calories, don't drink them!

Cereal sweep

Cereal packets can display misleading messages. Behind the promise of a nutritious start to the day is a cereal containing a lot of sugar. Take a good look at your cereal packets and see how much sugar they contain. A good breakfast cereal should contain hardly any sugar. It should be a useful source of fibre, not sugar.

Remember, you'll only crave sugar at breakfast if you don't get enough sleep, because your body interprets lack of sleep as an energy deficiency. You'll be tempted to meet these false energy demands with a cereal containing lots of sugar. Part of your Slim Habit is getting the right amount of sleep, so bin those sugary cereals. On your next shopping trip you'll be looking for a new cereal which is low in sugar and high in fibre.

No more sugary cereals!

Well Bread

What type of bread do you buy? Brown or wholemeal bread are the best options because they contain the most fibre. Why not white bread? Simply because it's had all the goodness taken out of it because it's made with refined flour. BUT the real danger is that most **commercial bread contains lots of salt. We get over 25% of our daily salt intake from bread**. As little as two medium slices of the worst example could contain 1 gram of salt, and **your RDA for salt is 6**.

Salt is needed in the baking process, but the reason there's so much in commercially-produced bread, buns and bagels is that salt increases shelf-life. It might shorten yours.

Don't buy bread where the salt content is not clearly marked 'per slice'. (You'll get a shock when you see how much salt is in each slice) Choose brown or wholemeal rather than white. If you want truly delicious bread, buy a bread maker. It'll save you money in the long run and you'll have delicious low-salt bread.

A slice is nice, but not too many!

Fridge and freezer secrets revealed

What do you notice about the contents of your fridge and freezer? How many ready meals have you got? Oven ready chips, frozen desserts, ice cream? Notice how much of what you have is fresh and how much is processed. What you actually eat may not be what you *think* you eat.

While you're looking at the labels, look for the amount of saturated fat and salt in the chips and ready meals. See how much sugar and fat there is in the ice cream and frozen desserts. **Now notice how little fibre they contain.**

There's nothing wrong with eating *some* processed food in the form of ready meals, but rather like alcohol, ready meals are best eaten in moderation. Why? Because as you'll notice, they contain high levels of salt, saturated fat and sugar, and almost **no fibre**. Remember that food companies deliberately remove fibre because it doesn't freeze well. **You need fibre**. Lack of fibre in your diet is a major cause of your evolutionary mismatch – and your weight gain.

Fresh out of fresh?

Lastly, how much fresh fruit and vegetables have you got? You may be surprised by how little you have – hopefully not! The thing to realise is that **fruit and vegetables contain fibre** as well as essential vitamins and minerals. Eating your 'five a day' is important, but what you eat should be fresh.

Beware of food companies who say that their processed food contains one or more of your 'five a day'. It might, but it certainly isn't fresh and it'll come with a whole lot of other ingredients you could do without. A 400g tin of Heinz tomato soup claims to be one of your 'five a day', but also contains 20 grams of sugar – that's 5 teaspoonfuls!

Fresh is good. The more fresh food you eat the better. Try having more fresh fruit during the day, it's a good habit to get into. Keep a bowl of fruit on the kitchen table and keep it well stocked.

Snacks, cookies, candy, cake n' things

Cakes are particularly high in sugar. An individual cup cake can contain as much as 16 grams of sugar, that's four teaspoons. That muffin you buy with your coffee in the morning can contain as much as 28 grams of sugar. That's over your RDA, so beware!

Snacks are designed to tempt you. Many contain a toxic temptation: a combination of fat and salt to nudge your preferences, and sugar and caffeine to get you on the hook.

Snacks deliver lots of unnecessary calories. If you eat a good breakfast which will reduce your hunger hormone ghrelin, you won't be stalked by hunger pangs throughout the day and feel the need to munch a chocolate bar. Snacks – sweet and savoury – should be occasional 'treats'- not a part of your diet. Best not to store them at home and avoid buying them during the day.

Snacks, an occasional treat, not part of your diet!

Preparation – let's go shopping

Before you do, consider this …

Your knowledge of food, and how much sugar, salt, fat and fibre it contains will get much better over the next few weeks. This will influence what you buy and change your diet to one that keeps within your RDAs. Good things will start to happen. Your insulin levels will improve and you'll move closer to getting back in sync with your evolutionary present. The secret is to experiment with new healthier foods and build up a list of things you enjoy eating, food that does you good, not harm.

Supermarkets are amazing …**but!** It's wise to remember that everything about the shopping experience has been designed to make you buy more. Walls of attractively-packaged processed food greet you. Carefully researched and designed algorithms manipulate and manage pricing. What you get on offer here, you pay for somewhere else. Offers and 'healthy options' are often designed to confuse rather than clarify, and they are masters of the science of product placement and layout. Supermarkets do a great job. They lure you in, and then direct your decision making.

Supermarkets also work very closely with food manufacturers. Together they work hard to produce processed food that tastes amazing, stimulates a sense of pleasure, and tempts greed. Much of it is food that requires the minimum of effort to prepare, attractively packaged to make sure it finds its way into your shopping basket. They are past masters at creating clever concoctions of ingredients, many of those ingredients, particularly sugar, in concentrations that are addictive or habit forming. These processed foods are deliberately designed to hook you so that you buy more …and more. This is where the best interests of supermarkets and food manufacturers and your best interests part company – and where your trust is betrayed.

If you're overweight or obese, the food industry conveniently shifts the blame onto you. You decide what you buy, it's your fault. The reality is that their processed foods are the cause of your evolutionary mismatch, which is why you weigh more than you would like, why you might not be as healthy as you would like to be – why the world has a obesity problem.

Food manufacturers spend millions promoting their brands to build confidence and get you to trust their products. Supermarkets fill their shelves with those brands, and trustingly, you buy them. You are being deceived, and that deception is affecting your weight – and your health.

Is it fair to expect that an iconic 400 gram tin of Heinz tomato soup should contain 5 teaspoons of sugar, that two slices of bread includes 16% of your daily allowance of salt, that a 500 ml bottle of cola contains 14 teaspoons of sugar, that a 415 gram can of baked beans contains 40% of your daily allowance of salt *and* 5 teaspoons of sugar? No it is not!

A new attitude to shopping

Food companies and supermarkets are not going to change their ways and governments are not going to make them. They might amend them when pressure mounts, but they won't do anything that will dent their sales or their profits. This is why it's important for you to build up your knowledge about the food you buy. **The only thing you should trust is your own – better informed – judgement.**

Here are some simple rules about shopping:

1. **Make a list before you go.** If you rely on the supermarket shelves to prompt your inspiration you'll buy things you don't need and be tempted to buy the wrong things. Know what you've got in the store cupboard and in the fridge. Plan your meals.

2. **Don't go shopping when you're hungry.** If you do, your basket will be full of sugary snacks and very little fresh food. **If you're hungry, drink a glass of water before you go.**

3. **Buy fresh FIRST.**

4. **Beware of foods that carry health claims**. Remember, 'low fat' can actually mean 'high fat' because sugar has been substituted for fat. Be highly suspicious of tins and cartons that claim to contain 'One of your five a day'. You only get full advantage from one of your 'five a day' from *fresh* **fruit and vegetables.**

5. **Avoid the aisles containing sugary drinks, fruit juices and smoothies.** They are all on the 'no buy' list.

6. **Become a food label expert**. Know your Recommended Daily Allowances – RDAs (sometimes known as an RI or Reference Intake) and know where to look for sugar, salt, total fat, saturated fat and fibre on the food label. Memorise these important RDAs:

TOTAL FAT	**70** grams
SATURATED FAT	**20** grams
SUGAR	**25** grams
FIBRE	**> 30** grams
SALT	**6** grams

You will find it a challenge to meet the sugar RDA of 25 grams, but it's in your interests to keep as near to it as you can.

Preparation – meals

One meal at a time

On your first shopping trip you might find it helpful to shop for one meal at a time. **Working out the RDAs one meal at a time might be a wise option**. It's up to you. You haven't started your programme yet so you have time and you're not under any pressure. It will give you time to research the supermarket shelves to see what you want to eat and consider the choices that are open to you.

Breakfast

You need to eat a good breakfast to kick start your energy-burning process and to reduce your hunger hormone ghrelin. Ideally, your breakfast should be at least a quarter of your daily food intake and **it should include protein**. Why protein? The main reason is because it'll make you feel less hungry. Cereal, toast and coffee will not do the trick.

What breakfast options would you like?

An example of a good breakfast which contains the three macro-nutrients protein, fat and carbohydrate plus fibre might be:
- A sugar-free, high-fibre cereal with milk and no added sugar.
- A piece of fruit. Where the skin is edible it should not be peeled. Eat the fruit separately or with your cereal.
- An egg in whatever way you prefer – fried, poached, scrambled, boiled, an omelette. Have it with ham, cheese or bacon.
- A slice of toast and butter.
- A cup of tea or coffee – preferably with no added sugar.

This is a standard breakfast, and one that will set you up for the day.

There are lots of other variations you can make. Vary your cereal, try porridge, add nuts to your cereal, try plain yogurt and mix it with fruit.

The total RDAs for the typical breakfast of cereal, fruit, egg and bacon, a slice of toast and butter, and a cup of tea or coffee are as follows:

	Grams	RDA
Total fat	30.5	70
Saturated fat	10.5	20
Sugar	12.1	25
Fibre	11	>30
Salt	1.4	6

*Tip: Learn to read the nutritional information on the food labels. You might find it useful to use a **nutrition app** like **Myfitnesspal**. This app, and others like it, will give you the nutritional information you want (the amount of total fat, saturated fat, sugar etc.,) for practically everything.*

Lunch

Ideally, it's better to have a **bigger lunch** and a smaller meal in the evening. You may be at work at lunchtime, which will mean you have to take care if you buy your lunch. Try eating as much fresh food as you can – this will keep you away from the high fat, high-salt meals. If you want something sweet, eat fruit. If you eat lunch at home or you take your lunch with you each day, have a rough plan of what you would like to eat and keep the total of your breakfast RDAs in the back of your mind.

Evening meal

Try and have this as early as possible. Remember if you eat a big meal late in the evening you'll be putting fuel into your boiler when it doesn't need it. Your blood sugar level will remain high which may affect your sleep patterns, and any excess energy will be stored as fat.

What's best, and what helps reduce fat, is to leave as long as you can between your evening meal and breakfast. 12 hours would be the ideal. In effect it's a mini fast. Oh, and **avoid after-dinner snacks and drinks**.

Your aim

Your aim at the end of each day is to have kept within your RDAs. Don't worry if you miss the target. Your RDAs are a guide. If you over-shoot, it's not the end of the world. The purpose of RDAs is to influence your choices and to guide you towards eating quality food in quantities that do not affect your biochemistry. Soon, keeping an eye on RDAs will become second nature, what you do – it will become a habit, a very good one.

It will all become clear

Over time new routines will emerge. A new shopping routine, a new mealtime routine. Your diet will change – for the better. You'll eat healthy, quality food. Most importantly, you'll eat what's good for you.

The choices you make will be *your informed choices*. You'll be able to discriminate between food that does you harm and good, healthy food. You'll be able to take back control of what you eat and how much you eat. You'll feel better about yourself and feel great too.

Eating out

Keeping to RDAs is not meant to kill off fun days and great evenings out. There'll be times when you go over the top and eat too much and your RDAs go out of the window. It doesn't matter as long as it only happens occasionally. You ought to bear a couple of things in mind though:

Fast food restaurants, are they off limits? No …BUT! It would be sensible if they were visited very rarely, and if you do you go, choose what you order with care. Have one course, make it the smallest size you can order, and DO NOT order a soda, a fruit juice or a smoothie. Water, tea or coffee is fine.

Most of what is sold in fast food restaurants is calorie-dense and **high in saturated fat, sugar and salt** – and that includes even some of their salad concoctions. The biggest problem is that you have absolutely no idea how many calories are in the meal you order, and that's what makes these restaurants a threat to your waistline, particularly if you're trying to lose weight and get your body back in sync.

More formal restaurants aren't quite such a problem because you have more choice and you can choose low-calorie options and limit what you order. If you're served big portions, don't feel obliged to eat everything on your plate. You can eat what you like, you're paying the bill remember!

If you think you've eaten too much on an evening out, make the next day a Low Calorie Day. It'll help reduce the effect of the extra calories.

Meal times

It's not always possible, but it's better if you can sit down – preferably not in front of the television or your computer – and take time to eat your meal. Why? Simply because you can concentrate on what you're eating, and how much you're eating. You don't want to rush your meals, which it's easy to do if you're concentrating on something else. You have to give your satiety signal time to work. Remember the hormone PYY in your small intestine that tells you when you've eaten enough? It won't have had time to be activated by the food you're eating if you eat too quickly. Eat too quickly and you'll eat too much. **It takes 20 minutes for your PYY signal to be activated. Take time to enjoy your food.**

Ready meals

Ready meals answer a need in a busy workaday world. Convenient and tasty, they can make life easier – but at a price. The level of total fat, saturated fat, sugar and salt in many of these meals are at levels that do you positive harm when you eat too many of them. Most important of all, they contain very little fibre. Food manufacturers have removed it because fibre doesn't freeze well. You'll soon find that the RDAs on ready meals will put you over your RDA limit very quickly. Avoid eating ready meals as much as you can.

New habits, a new beginning

The discipline of keeping within your RDAs might take a little time to get used to, but as you progress, your knowledge about food products will grow. You'll become aware of what is good and what is bad, and because you've done your homework, the choices you make will be informed choices. You'll be more particular about what you eat, you'll find that you eat new and interesting foods – that do you good, not harm. Your waistline will get smaller, and you'll get healthier.

Preparation – four new habits

There are four essential habits you need to learn. It might be a good idea to start learning them now, before your start date. **It takes a minimum of 21 days for you to learn a new habit, for it to become 'hot-wired' in your brain,** so the sooner you start the better.

The Sleep Habit

Your new habit: Sleep between 7 and 7½ hours every night.

Why do you need to get this amount of sleep? Because if you get less, and particularly if you consistently get less than 7–7½ hours, your metabolism won't function properly, and **your body will interpret lack of sleep as an energy deficiency.** You'll produce more grehlin and less leptin, and be tempted to eat a sugary breakfast when you get up to boost your energy level. It'll then become difficult to keep the lid on the urge to snack during the day. The consequence of not getting the right amount of sleep is weight gain.

What to do:

1. Get into the habit of going to bed early. This may mean changing well-established routines and informing family members of your intentions.

2. Eat your evening meal as early as you can. It's best if this is a small meal rather than a large one. You don't need a lot of food in the evening. Any excess energy you take on board late is likely to be stored as fat.

3. Don't have any late evening snacks, sweet drinks or alcohol. If you do, your blood sugar level will remain high and you'll find sleep difficult.

4. Don't drink coffee after your evening meal. Coffee can reduce the secretion of your sleep-inducing hormone melatonin by up to 50%, so getting to sleep might not be easy.

5. Don't look at a screen, be it a TV, phone, iPad or laptop at least an hour before you go to bed. If you do your brain will think it's still daylight and getting to sleep may be difficult.

6. Make sure your bedroom is as dark as it can be. You will get a better sleep if your room is dark and not illuminated by electrical alarm clocks / radios etc.

When you start taking exercise you'll find one of the benefits is that exercise will help you get a good night's sleep.

The Drink Water Habit

Your new habit: To drink 7–8 glasses of water each day

Drinking 7–8 glasses of water a day will keep you properly hydrated, reduce any bloating and keep all your biochemical processes working properly – and help you to lose weight.

Drinking the right amount of water is just question of getting into a routine and choosing to drink water rather than anything else.

Try this as a starter routine: (you can adjust it to suit your day)
- A glass when you wake up or half an hour before breakfast
- One glass before you start work or at about 9.30
- A glass at 11.00
- 30 minutes before lunch – 12.30
- One at about 4pm
- A glass before you leave work – 5pm
- A glass half an hour before dinner – 6.30pm
- A glass about 8pm

When you first start you will find that you'll visit the bathroom a bit more often, but your bladder will adjust over time and your visits will become less frequent.

Remember! Hunger and thirst signals are easily confused. If you feel a hunger pang, answer it with a glass of water, not with food.

The No Snack Habit

Your new habit: Cut out snacks.

If you eat three good meals a day, you don't answer thirst signals with food, and you get a good night's sleep, you probably won't feel the need to snack, so this habit maybe easier than you imagine.

Snacking is a habit, and a very dangerous one. If you're a regular 'snacker' you're probably getting a third of your calories from snacks.

Whether it's a delicious chocolate bar or a super sugary fruit juice, snacks play a huge part in messing up your biochemical processes.

If you feel hungry the first thing to do is to have a drink of water. If you still feel hungry have a piece of fruit.

Snacks? Just give them a miss!

The Small Portion Habit

Your new habit: Reduce your portion sizes.

It's very easy to eat too much. Most of us do – sometimes without noticing. In a lot of cases it all comes down to how much you put on your plate – or how much a restaurant puts on your plate. We all need to eat less, and a very good way of doing this is to reduce your portion sizes. Don't fill your plate with food. If you're eating out don't accept a mountain of food, no matter how tempting.

The best way to make sure you reduce your portion sizes is to eat off a small plate. Don't pile up your food on your plate, and avoid second helpings. When you eat out ask for a small portion or just don't eat everything that's put in front of you. **It's not waste when it comes to your waist.**

This is such a simple habit, but one that can make a huge difference.

Remember, practice these habits every day for 21 days and you'll find that they become part of your routine, of what you do, second nature.

Your diet – ready to go?

Your Diet preparation should have been a period of discovery. You'll have become aware of what you've been eating, which may or may not have been a surprise to you. Whatever the case you'll also have become aware of the amount of fat, saturated fat, sugar, salt and fibre that was in your diet.

Getting to grips with food labels and RDAs takes a bit of getting used to, but with practice you'll find it easy, particularly as you become more familiar with your new shopping habits and food preferences.

Take as much time as you need to finish your preparation. When you think you've done all you need to do, set a date to start **Your Slim Habit.** Now it's time to prepare for your Low Calorie Days and your exercise programme.

Preparation – Low Calorie Days

There are two important things you need to do in preparation for your **Low Calorie Days.**

1. Work out a selection of Low Calorie Day meals.

2. Understand how to use Low Calorie Days

Low Calorie Day Meals

Low Calorie Days are days when you eat no more than 550 calories. This is the only time on the Slim Habit programme that you concentrate on the number of calories you eat, so it's a good idea to research and plan what you intend to eat on Low Calorie Days.

What you **don't** want to do on a Low Calorie Day is worry about counting calories. Your life will be much simpler if you know in advance the calorie values of things you would like to eat, and you have worked out what you want your daily menu to look like. It's a good idea to add variety to keep things interesting.

550 calories doesn't give you much scope for creating culinary masterpieces, and it's perhaps wise not to try. Low Calorie Days are not the best days to tease your senses with tempting aromas. The secret is to keep things simple, certainly in the beginning. Later on if you feel that you want to be more adventurous on your Low Calorie Days then there are endless possibilities. Try making three or four Low Calorie Day menus and alternate them. There are some simple menu suggestions along with calorie counts on page 152.

What to expect …

You might be a little anxious at the thought of not eating very much, but you'll soon get used to it. **Make sure you always start the day with a good breakfast that includes both protein and carbohydrate**. Protein will make you feel less hungry. Why not go to work on an egg?

As the day progresses, especially in the late afternoon, you may be surprised that you are not feeling particularly hungry. You might also notice you're in a better mood. Reducing your calorie intake can have a positive effect on your mood, which is a useful bonus when you're trying to get used to Low Calorie Days.

Low Calorie Days will not only put you in a better mood, they'll make you feel good. They're doing you good too. Not only will **you lose weight without losing muscle**, you'll have the ability to take control of your weight. There are other benefits too. It allows your body time for your repairs and maintenance genes to get to work. It's good for the health of your heart, your insulin sensitivity, it reduces the chance of you getting type 2 diabetes …and **importantly, it reconnects you to your evolutionary present and gets you back in sync.** Your body starts to work *with* you rather than being unable to work *for* you.

Deciding your Low Calorie Day frequency

Here's a guide to how to use Low Calorie days.

One day per week: Do one day on your first week. Use a one-day LCD after you've achieved your target weight as a way of keeping yourself in sync and to allow your body to rest and repair.

Two days per week: Two LCDs per week will get you back in sync and is the best way to achieve long-term sustainable weight loss. This is the most common approach to weight loss using LCDs.

Three days per week: You will lose more weight on three LCDs a week. If you decide to go down this route, you might find that it's easier to do a three-day regime every other week rather than every week.

Every other day: This is quite a 'full on' approach to weight loss and you should exercise caution when deciding on this option. Certainly it would be wise to do it on alternate weeks if it's what you decide to do.

Low Calorie Days are never done on consecutive days

> *Tip: A Low Calorie Day is always useful following a day when you've eaten more than you should. It gets you back to where you were. Yes, you can enjoy yourself and still be in control of your weight!*

What about normal days?

On normal days, there is no restriction on what you eat. All you have to do is to keep as near as you can to your RDA of sugar, fibre, salt, fat and saturated fat. What you want to avoid doing after a Low Calorie Day is to make up for lost ground and eat more. This shouldn't be a problem because you'll find that you don't feel hungry after a Low Calorie Day, particularly at the start of the day.

Be patient

When you first start, the thought of eating very little for a whole day can be a little daunting, but when you've done it once or twice you'll think nothing of it. If you include protein in what you eat for breakfast it will help stave off any hunger pangs and you probably won't feel like eating until lunchtime.

Weight loss will be gradual, but it will be genuine weight loss. It'll be fat loss and virtually no muscle loss, unlike a diet where you lose roughly the same amount of muscle as you do fat.

When you keep within your RDAs and do Low Calorie Days you'll find it's a winning combination especially when taken with exercise …

Preparation – exercise

Your approach to exercise

The changes you are about to make to your life, will have a hugely positive effect on your life and your general health. The one thing which will supercharge your efforts is …exercise.

How you approach exercise may colour how much benefit you get from it. Exercise should never be a chore, but something you enjoy and look forward to. It's important to look upon exercise as a benefit, something that will support your efforts to lose weight, help to reduce stress and get you back in sync – *and* improve your health.

Taking regular exercise can give you an amazing feeling of achievement. You'll feel better – and better about yourself. Don't think about it as a chore, just make a conscious effort to include exercise as a part of what you do, and yes, it'll soon become a habit.

There are three types of exercise you need to take: aerobic, resistance and flexibility. There is a complete section titled 'Exercise for you' on page 119. Read it before you start. Here you will learn what to do and get advice on how to set up your own exercise programme. It's simple and easy to do.

You might also find it helpful to use visualisation. It will help you to get started and make it easier for you to meet your exercise goals.

Remember, exercise won't be a chore if you do it regularly and it becomes part of your life. The more you do the fitter you'll be, and the more enjoyable it will become.

Preparation – weight and measure

Setting your base line

Before you start your Slim Habit you need to establish your base line. You need to know what you weigh **and** what you measure so that you can judge your progress. So, get some reliable scales, a tape measure, and a note book.

Weight

It's always best to weigh yourself at the same time every day. It's a good idea to weigh yourself as soon as you get up in the morning. How often you weigh yourself is up to you, but expect your weight to fluctuate from day to day. You will lose a pleasing amount of weight after a Low Calorie Day, for example, but some of that weight will return the following day. Over time, the trend will be down.

Measurements

As your weight fluctuates from day to day, measuring yourself gives you a better indication of how much progress you are making.

When you first start you may be pleasantly surprised by how much weight you lose. Much of this will be retained water. This loss will be reflected on the scales *and* in your measurements. However, when you start to exercise and gain more muscle, your scales won't give you an accurate picture of your actual fat loss because muscle weighs more that fat. If you measure yourself it will confirm that you *are* making progress.

Measure yourself on your start date to set your base line and then thereafter once a week.

Here's what you should measure:
- **Waist:** Just above the hipbone.
- **Hips:** From the centre of your bottom, round to just above the pubic bone.
- **Thighs:** Centre or largest part of your thigh.
- **Calf:** Round the middle of your calf.
- **Biceps:** Half way between your elbow and your armpit.

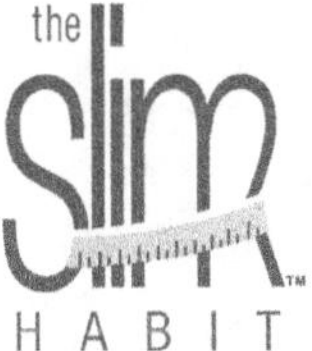

Part Three

What You Need To Do

This is *your* Slim Habit. This is your chance to set a new course, to take back control of your weight and enjoy a healthy life.

You have the knowledge!

Now you know what causes your evolutionary mismatch and why your biochemistry is able to take control of why you eat and what you eat. There is no longer any mystery of why things happen, and now you know what you can do to make real and lasting change in your life. **Knowledge is power and you have that power.**

Diet – Recommended Daily Allowances

Keep as near to your Recommended Daily Allowances as you can and you will get your body back in sync with your evolutionary present. Your biochemistry will work *for* you, rather than *against* you.

Low Calorie Days

Low Calorie days give you the ability to manage and control your weight and to keep your body in sync, trim and healthy.

Exercise

Regular aerobic, resistance and flexibility exercise will supercharge your weight loss and allow you to enjoy a slim healthy life.

The Slim Habit is:

Knowledge
Diet – Recommended Daily Allowances
Low Calorie Days
Exercise

Your Slim Habit

If you've completed the preparation phrase, you should be ready to start your Slim Habit. Remember, your Slim Habit is not like a diet. It's not something you do for a few weeks. It's a new way of life. The Slim Habits you learn will become part of what you do, of who you are. Its secret is its simplicity. All you have to do is to try, to be determined, and success will be yours. This is the moment when you take control.

Weight and Measure

On Day One, weigh and measure yourself at the beginning of the day before your first meal. This is your base line.

Date	
WEIGHT	
WAIST	
HIPS	
THIGHS	
CALF	
BICEPS	

Weigh yourself as often as you like. It's best you weigh yourself at the beginning of the day before breakfast, but remember that your weight will fluctuate. Best to record your weight at the end of each week as well as taking your measurements.

Weekly routine

One week at a time. At the beginning of each week you need to take three decisions. About your diet, how many Low Calorie Days you will do, and the exercise you will take. These decisions will be your guide for the week.

Decision 1 – Diet

Decide on a menu plan for the first week. This will help you to get more familiar with RDAs, make shopping easier and increase your food awareness.

Continue to plan your meals for as long as you think necessary. You can stop the detailed planning once you feel confident that you have built up sufficient knowledge of RDAs. Selecting what to buy takes a little time, matching up what you would like to eat with your RDAs, but the whole process, and particularly RDA awareness, becomes easy to do the more you do it. It's just a new habit to learn. It will soon become second nature.

A sample meal plan for a breakfast might look like this:

BREAKFAST	Total fat (70g)	Saturated Fat (20g)	Sugar (25g)	Fibre (>30g)	Salt (6g)
Cereal with skimmed milk and blueberries	2	1	6	11	2.05
1 × boiled egg	14	4			
Toast, butter	5	3	1	2	0.4
Coffee and skimmed milk			1		0.25
Total Grams	21	8	9	13	2.7

> *Tip: Recommended Daily Allowances are a guide. If you exceed them from time to time — but not excessively — it's not the end of the world. Your efforts to lose weight and improve your health will not be compromised forever. **What is important** is that you are aware of what RDAs are, and that you do your best to keep as near to the them as possible.*

Decision 2 – Low Calorie Days

Decide on how many Low Calorie Days you will do each week and the days you intend to do them. Make that decision at the beginning of each week and then keep to your schedule.

Week 1 should be one day. Thereafter two Low Calorie Days a week will deliver the gradual and lasting weight loss you want. Add another day if you feel confident enough to do so. Low Calorie Days on alternate days will improve results, but it's best to do this on alternate weeks. Remember, you are after long-lasting, gradual weight loss. Patience and persistence produces the best results.

It's a good idea to decide which days are best for you to have a Low Calorie Day. You might find that one weekday and one day at the weekend might suit you best. A routine of the same days each week might be an easier option so that you don't forget. Whatever you decide, try out different combinations during the first three weeks until you get yourself into a routine. Make a chart or make a diary entry to make sure you don't miss a Low Calorie Day.

	Sun	Mon	Tues	Wed	Thur	Fri	Sat
Week 1	LCD						
Week 2		LCD			LCD		
Week 3			LCD			LCD	
Week 4				LCD			LCD

Decision 3 – Exercise

Decide at the beginning of each week what exercise you are going to do and when you are going to do it. Exercise is easy to put off, so it's a good idea to decide what you are going to do, to have a weekly plan, and keep to it. It doesn't have to be cast in stone, but if you get into the habit of deciding what you are going to do at the beginning of each week, you'll get into a routine and you'll get your exercise done. There are exercise plans in the *Exercise for You* section.

Remember, there are three types of exercise you need to do:

1. **Aerobic**, which in the *Exercise for You* plan involves **walking**. No, you're not going to be asked to train to run a marathon, but just to get moving and get your heart beating a little faster with regular aerobic exercise.

2. **Resistance**, which involves using weights three times a week.

3. **Flexibility**, which is stretching.

Exercise will turbocharge your weight loss and significantly improve your general health.

Your Four New Habits

If you've already started these new habits, so much the better. Within 21 days of starting these new habits they'll become second nature to you. These are very simple habits, but vitally important. The benefits are huge – best of all they'll make you feel great.

> **1. The Sleep Habit – Get between 7 & 7½ hours sleep every day.**

This habit will involve your changing usual routine. It may take a bit of getting used to, but the pay-off is worth it. Remember to eat your evening meal as early as you can, avoid late night snacks or alcoholic drinks and be determined not to look at your computer/iPad/phone at least an hour before you turn in. The quality of your sleep is as important as the length of your sleep.

> **2. The No Snack Habit – Cut out snacks.**

You don't need to snack. Snacks are an invention designed by food companies to get you to buy more of their products. It's estimated that 25% of our daily calorie intake comes from snacks. Don't give in to temptation. If you feel hungry drink a glass of water. If you still feel hungry eat a piece of fruit.

> **3. The Drink Water Habit – Drink between 7–8 glasses a day.**

It's in the best interests of your health and your metabolism to be properly hydrated. Your metabolism works best when you are. You avoid becoming bloated when you're properly hydrated.

You've probably been answering thirst signals with food. Drinking water regularly throughout the day will help prevent that. You'll get used to drinking more water and feel much better for it – and it'll help you lose weight too.

4. The Small Portion Habit – Reduce your portion sizes.

This is the simplest way to stop eating too much. Reduce your portion sizes and you'll reduce your weight. Say no to second helpings. You'll find that the less you eat the less you want to eat. Use a small plate if you think it might help.

And success comes from...commitment!

You now know why things happen. You have the knowledge and the tools to put them right. Your weight, your health is now in your hands.

The Slim Habit is simple, but effective. All it requires is your commitment, a commitment to change your habits and to maintain those habits. Just remember that the Slim Habit is not a diet, it's not something you do for a while and then stop, even when you've reached your target weight. It's a means to achieve a better, slimmer, healthier life – a commitment for life. The habits you have learned will become hard-wired in your brain, and will continue to support your new slim, healthy life. You may wish to adjust what you do from time to time, like the number of Low Calorie Days you do each week, for example, but the ongoing management of your weight and your health is down to you. You know how to do it. Just do it!

Your Slim Habit – make it work for you.

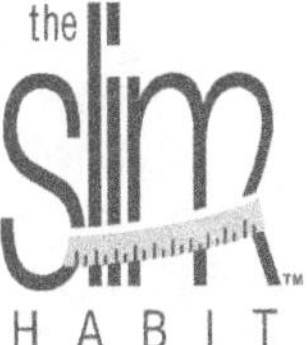

Part Four

Exercise For You

Exercise will supercharge your efforts to lose weight, get your body back into balance and keep you slim and healthy. Exercise isn't something you should think of as a chore. Put your mind to it and it'll be enjoyable and rewarding.

Finding time for exercise can be a problem. We all lead very busy lives. There's always too much to do. People and events seem to have a constant demand on our time. Of course it can be difficult to fit exercise into your busy routine, but it's essential that you do.

The exercises The Slim Habit suggests you do are very easy. Once you get started and get into them, they'll become a part of what you do, part of your daily routine. Don't be surprised to find yourself looking for ways of doing more exercise and increasing your fitness once the benefits start to come through.

There are three types of exercise you need to take: aerobic, resistance and flexibility.

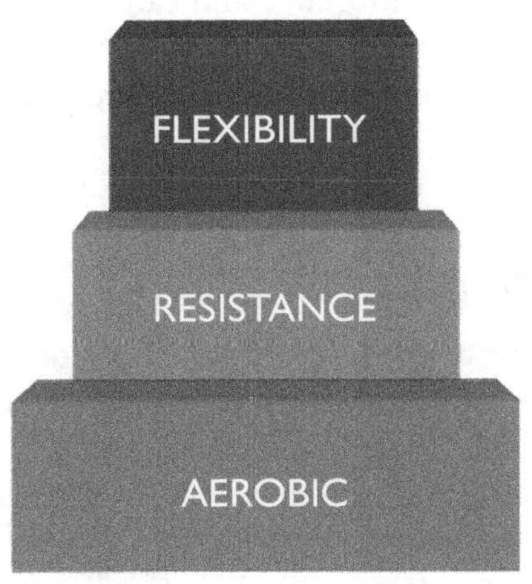

Exercise Preparation

Before you start, you need to do a little preparation!

Medical

If you suffer from any medical condition, or if you have any concerns *at all*, you should see your doctor before you start any weight loss or exercise program. This is particularly important if you have heart disease, high blood pressure, or you show any cardiovascular risk factors. If in doubt – ask.

Get the right kit

You don't have to spend a fortune on new exercise kit, but you do need a few essentials. Buy a good pair of trainers or walking shoes – you need to cushion your joints while you're exercising.

Dress so that you feel comfortable and can move comfortably. Don't wear clothes that make you too hot, and don't wear too little and get cold. Dress appropriately for the temperature and the exercise you're going to do.

Make time for exercise

When are you going to do your exercise? If you don't think about this, you'll get to the end of a day and find you've run out of time to do it. You might find it helpful in the beginning if you draw up a timetable. Write down what you're going to do and when you're going to do it. It'll only take you a few minutes to do this. Once your exercises are part of your daily routine you can probably dispense with timetables.

Safety

When you exercise, please think about safety. If you're walking or running, face the oncoming traffic. Make sure you can be seen, especially at night. Wear bright or reflective clothing. If you're riding a bike, wear a helmet. Take note of the weather and dress appropriately.

Steady as she goes

In your enthusiasm, DO NOT rush out and over-do it. Build up *slowly* and *gradually*. If you overdo it in the beginning, you'll pay the price and lose your enthusiasm. You *will* achieve your goal if you are sensible and determined.

Drink

Make sure you don't get dehydrated. Drink plenty of water before you start your exercise, and again after you've finished.

Eating

Don't go and eat a large meal immediately after you've finished a session of deliberate walking. If you do, you'll give your heart too much to do. Let it deal with looking after your muscles first. Leave at least an hour after exercising before eating a large meal.

Not when you're ill

If you've got a cold or a fever, or you're feeling 'under the weather', *don't exercise. Listen to your body.* When you're better, don't rush back at full intensity. If you resume gradually, you'll get back to where you left off more quickly.

Respect injuries

If you injure yourself, don't try to exercise until the injured part is completely better. It'll take longer to heal if you don't. Find another exercise which avoids aggravating your injury. **Do NOT "work through pain"**.

Listen to your body

Notice, listen and pay attention – when your body speaks to you, please take note! Learn to notice the difference between your body complaining about being given some unexpected or new exercise, and a genuine warning. If your muscles have not been exercised for some time, they'll complain. That's not usually anything to worry about. If you're in any doubt, see your doctor.

Aerobic exercise

Aerobic exercise, sometimes referred to as cardiovascular exercise, is the exercise that speeds up your heart rate and gets your metabolism going. It includes exercise like walking, running and bicycling. Aerobic exercise is important because it burns fat. It helps to reduce stress. It oxygenates. It makes you healthier and helps to protect you from heart disease and stroke. In terms of weight loss and reducing stress levels and improving your general health, of the three types of exercise you will be doing, *aerobic exercise is by far the most important.*

Time to get moving

The aerobic exercise The Slim Habit recommends is – **walking**. Walking will give you all the aerobic exercise you need. There's no need to join a gym, spend lots of money on special clothing or get a personal trainer. All you need to do is to be able to measure how much walking you do. You need to get a simple pedometer or something like a Fitbit that will tell you how many paces you take.

Getting started

When you first start to take regular exercise, it's wise to start gradually and build up. Here are the progressions that will deliver the results you want.

Your daily target is 10,000 paces!

10,000 paces may sound a lot, but you'll be surprised how many steps you take just doing routine chores around the house or at work.

Over a period that you feel comfortable with, work up to 5,000 paces. Once you've achieved that, move up to 7,500 and then 10,000. If you can do more, so much the better. 10,000 paces should be your daily minimum. This is a good level of aerobic exercise.

Deliberate walking

To increase your level of fitness once you are achieving 10,000 paces a day, you can progress to 'deliberate walking'. Deliberate walking is just another way of describing walking at a faster pace. As a guide, this might be between **120 and 130 paces a minute**. Try and do deliberate walking three times a week. It can be part of your 10,000 paces if you like, or you can do more.

Start by doing 10 minutes three times each week and then work up to 30 minutes three times each week.

Your walking habit

Having a daily target will get you to adopt better, healthier habits. Maybe you'll walk up the stairs rather than take the lift, walk to the shops rather than take the car, walk some of the way to work, use your lunch break to go for a walk. The discipline of your new walking habit will be life-changing – and it's so simple to do.

Resistance exercise

Resistance exercise is training with weights, and using specific exercises without weights, to build muscle and improve muscle strength. It helps to improve your metabolism. Healthy muscle burns more calories and helps to reduce fat. You have 620 muscles in your body. The more 'tuned' they are, the more efficiently you function, and the healthier you are.

Resistance exercise also helps your bones. Bones are active living tissues. New bone tissue is constantly being formed, and old tissue absorbed. Resistance exercise puts your bones under what might be called 'useful' stress. This helps to *stimulate bone formation* – and when you consider that we lose 0.5% of bone mass every year over the age of 40, this is very important because it keeps your bones healthy and strong.

Resistance exercise will also help to improve your cholesterol levels, and reduce your blood pressure. As an extra bonus, it will improve your posture and help you to look good.

As you get older – beyond the age of 35 – resistance training becomes even more important. Every ten years your metabolic rate will reduce by *up to 5%*. In other words, the older you become, the less efficient your body will be at burning calories. If you take no exercise at all, you're likely to experience an increase in weight of up to 15 pounds in a ten-year period. Much of this is because of a loss of muscle tissue, which often translates into an increase in body fat. If you can maintain both your muscle mass and strength by resistance training, you'll be going a long way to maintaining an efficient metabolic rate and avoiding unwanted weight gain.

It's never too late to do this. Previously it was thought that muscle degeneration was an irreversible process: however, a recent Canadian study showed that this is not the case. Regular resistance training can *reverse* signs of ageing in muscles – a powerful reason why the exercise you take throughout your life should include resistance training.

Resistance training is an essential part of your exercise regime. It increases your endurance, and most important of all, it promotes weight loss and makes you feel better.

15 minutes three times a week!

This is all you need to do to tone up your muscles and improve your metabolism. Of course you can do more, and the fitter you become the more you will want to do.

Before you start resistance exercises

First, find a space where you can do your exercises safely and in peace.

Weights

When you buy your weights, don't buy heavy ones that you can only just lift. If you start with heavy weights, all you'll do is injure yourself. *It's not the weight that's important, but the number of repetitions you do. It's the number of repetitions which burns off the fat.* Get weights that you feel comfortable with. Take advice when you buy them. Start with a weight that feels almost too light. It will feel much heavier the more repetitions you do. You can always progress to a heavier weight later on.

Repetitions and sets

When doing an exercise involving weights, *'High repetition, low weight' will get you the best results.* The idea is to repeat each exercise until you find you can't do any more – without straining. Initially you may find that you can only manage 5 repetitions, but don't be discouraged by this. Make 5 repetitions the number of repetitions in the set for this exercise and then repeat the set. As you progress you can change the number of repetitions in each set if you wish – or just repeat the set.

Always rest between each set of repetitions. Flex your muscles a little. When you lift your weights, don't jerk them. Don't lock your joints. Lift your weight slowly and gently, and lower it in a similar way. When doing an exercise not using weights slowly build up the number of repetitions you do in each set.

Breathing

How you breathe when you take exercise is very important. Don't hold your breath when you lift your weights. Breathe naturally: *exhale* when you lift your weight, and *inhale* when you lower your weight.

48 hours

You should leave *48 hours* in between every resistance training session. This will allow your muscles to recover, and give you optimum weight loss. Resistance exercises will build up your muscle and burn fat. These exercises have been put together so that you can do them at home. No great expense is required. All you'll need is a set of weights and you're ready to go.

Just remember…

- Each exercise should be done in sets of repetitions: for example, two sets of eight repetitions. The number of sets and repetitions will vary for each exercise.

- You should always rest between each set.

- You should always leave 48 hours between resistance exercise sessions to allow your muscles to recover.

- High-repetition, low-resistance exercise is what you should aim for. When you start the exercise, the first few repetitions will not feel difficult, but as you progress they will become increasingly more difficult. Later on, you will find that you'll be able to gradually increase the number of repetitions you do in each set before you start to feel tired.

- Each exercise set should be performed in a set of between eight and fifteen repetitions.

- If you are comfortable doing one set of repetitions, add another. In time, you'll be able to reach 3–4 sets per exercise. Once you can do this, you may wish to increase the weight you're lifting.

- Warm up before you begin to exercise. Do some stretching exercises.

- Fill your 15 minutes of resistance exercises with different exercises – see the examples illustrated. Vary the exercises each session.

Some 'Do's and Don'ts' about how to use weights:

- Don't lock your joints.

- Don't jerk the weight when you lift it.

- Don't hold your breath. Breathe *out* when you lift the weight, breathe *in* when you lower the weight.

- If you're standing, keep your feet hip-width apart and your knees slightly bent.

- Lift the weight slowly and smoothly.

Exercise 1
LEGS, HIPS AND KNEES

Begin
1.   Stand with your feet approximately 18 inches (45cms) apart.
2.   Hold a weight in each hand down by your side, palms towards your body.

Action
1.   Bend your knees slowly and lower yourself approximately 10 inches (25cms).
2.   Keep your arms by your side.
3.   Slowly stand up straight again.
4.   Start with 8 reps per set.

Notice!
1.   Your back should remain straight.
2.   Your arms should remain straight down by your side. Don't allow them to move forward.

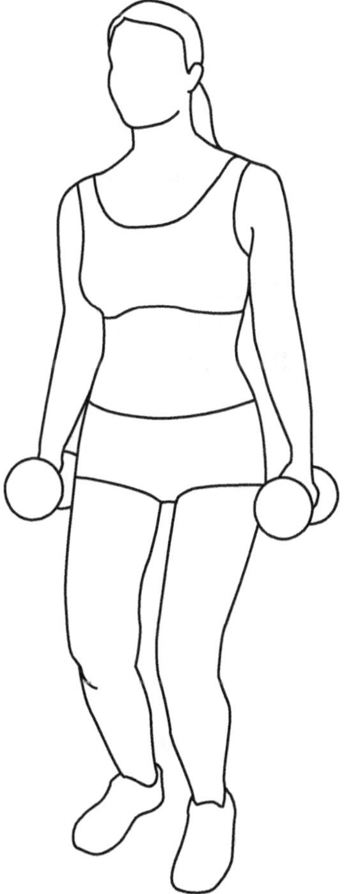

Exercise 2
CALVES, FEET AND ANKLES

Begin
1. You need to support yourself whilst standing, so either hold on to the back of a chair, or face a wall and place your palms flat on the wall, arms stretched, but not locked.
2. Your feet should be approximately 18 inches (45cms) apart.

Action
1. Slowly raise yourself onto your toes.
2. Hold that position for 5 seconds.
3. Lower yourself down again.
4. Start with 8 to 10 reps per set.

Notice!
1. Your back should remain straight.
2. Remember not to lock your knees.

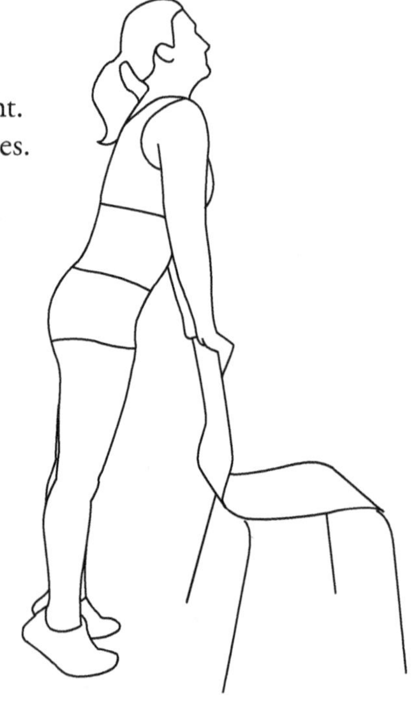

Exercise 3
HIPS, BUTTOCKS AND THIGHS

Begin
1. You will need a strong chair. The seat should be firm and the height of the seat should be normal.
2. Stand approximately 12 inches (30cms) directly in front of the chair.
3. Your feet should be approximately 18 (45cms) inches apart.
4. Hold your arms out in front of you, palms down.
5. Lean forward very slightly from your waist.

Action
1. With your weight on your heels, slowly lower yourself down so that you are almost sitting on the chair. Don't sit down.
2. Slowly stand back up again.
3. Start with 8 reps per set.

Notice
1. Keep your arms straight out in front of you.
2. Keep your head upright and look straight ahead.

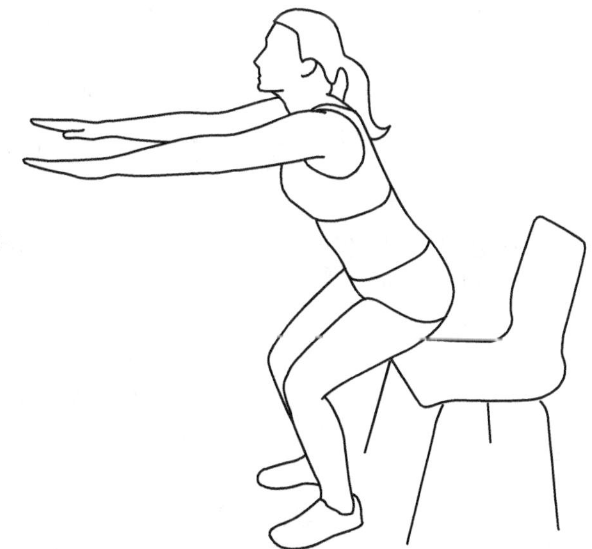

Exercise 4
UPPER BACK, SHOULDERS AND ARMS

Begin
1. Sit down on a chair.
2. Don't lean back and keep your back straight.
3. Keep your feet approximately 18 inches (45cms) apart.
3. Hold a weight in each hand.
4. Let your arms hang down either side of the chair.

Action
1. Lift both hands slowly to the top of your chest allowing the weight to rotate 90°, knuckles forward.
2. Lower the dumbbell slowly to the starting position.
3. Do this again, this time keep your palms forward as you raise the weights.
4. Try 15 reps per set.

Notice!
1. Keep upright and look straight in front of you.
2. Bring both weights up at the same time. Exhale as you lift.

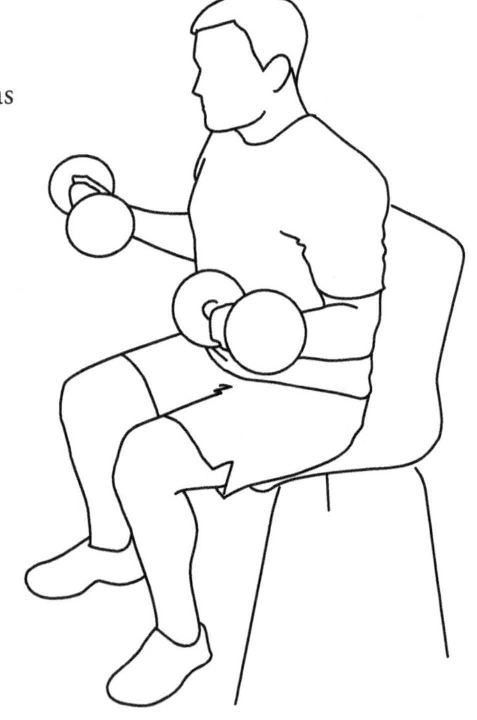

Exercise 5
UPPER BACK, SHOULDERS AND ARMS

Begin
1. Stand with your legs approximately 18 inches (45cms) apart.
2. Hold a weight in each hand, palms facing inwards.

Action
1. Lift both weights simultaneously to shoulder level, keeping your elbows out.
2. Lower the weights slowly to the start position.
3. Repeat. Do between 8 and 15 reps per set.

Notice!
1. When the weights are at shoulder height, try to keep your elbows parallel to the ground.

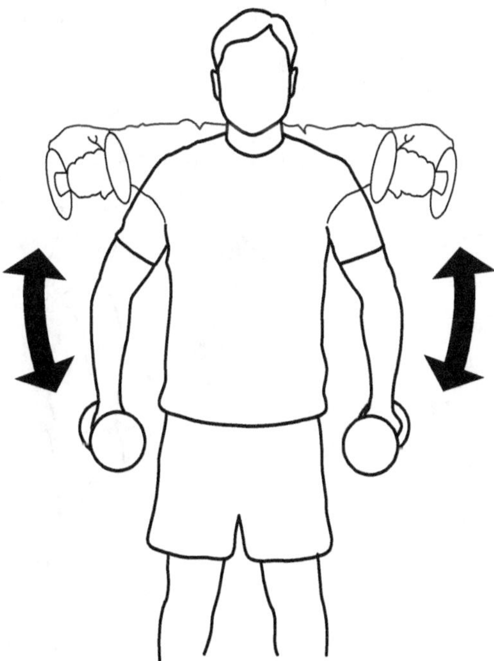

Exercise 6
ARMS, SHOULDERS AND UPPER BACK

Begin
1. Stand with your feet approximately 18 inches (45cms) apart.
2. Hold a weight in each hand, palms facing inwards.

Action
1. Keeping your arms straight, lift both weights slowly until they are parallel with the floor.
2. Slowly lower the weights to the starting position.
3. Do between 6 and 12 reps per set.

Notice!
1. Don't lock your knees. Keep them slightly bent.
2. Keep your elbows straight.

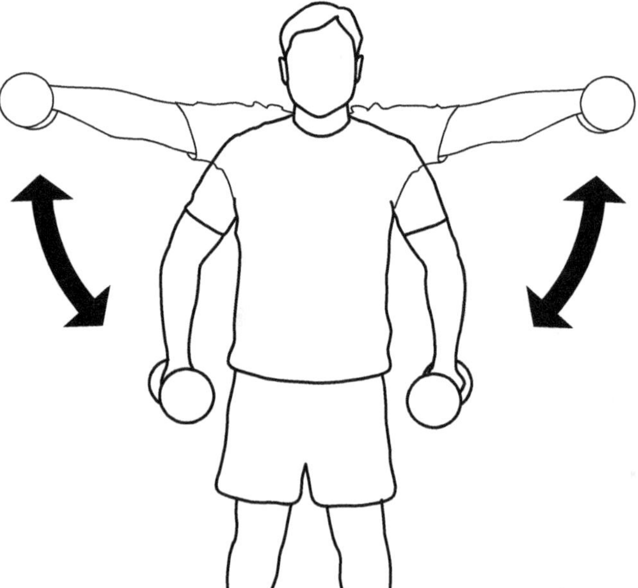

Exercise 7
ARM EXERCISE – BICEPS

Begin
1. Sit on a chair or bench with your legs quite wide apart.
2. Hold a weight in your left hand, palm facing upwards.
3. Rest your left elbow on your inside knee.
4. Place your right hand on the top of your right knee.

Action
1. Bring the weight up slowly, curling towards your shoulder.
2. Slowly lower the weight to the starting position.
3. Now transfer the weight to your right hand and repeat the exercise.
3. Try 6 to 12 reps per arm, per set.

Notice!
1. Keep your elbow tight to your knee.
2. Lean slightly forward. Don't lean backwards.

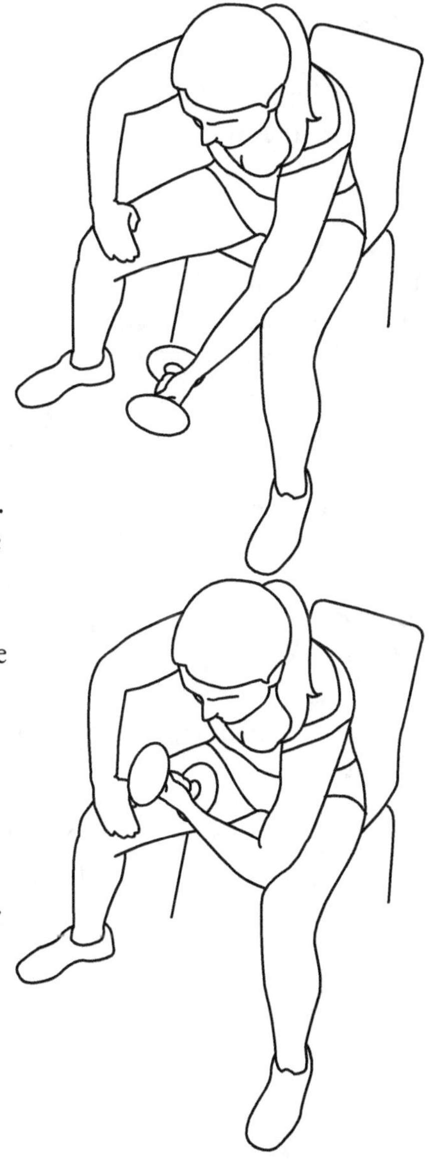

Exercise 8
ARM EXERCISE – TRICEPS

Begin
1. Sit on a chair or a bench.
2. Hold one end of a weight with both hands.
3. Raise the weight above your head.

Action
1. Slowly lower the weight behind your head until you feel your arm muscles tightening.
2. Raise the weight back to the starting position above your head and stretch your arms.
3. Do between 6 and 12 reps per set.

Notice!
1. Don't do this exercise with a weight which is too heavy.
2. Keep your back straight when you are doing this exercise.

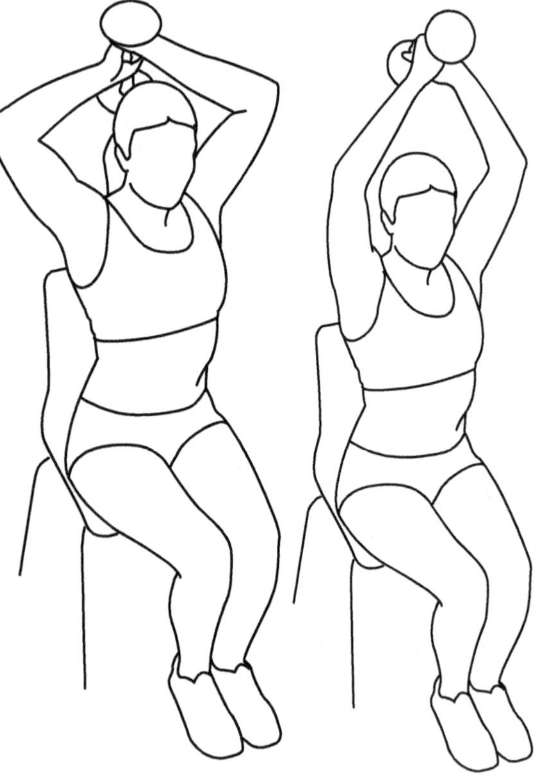

Exercise 9
ABDOMINALS – TOP

Begin
1. Lie flat on the floor.
2. Bend your knees, keeping your feet together.
3. Now lift your knees so that they are over your hips.
4. Place your fingers at the side of your head as if you are saluting with both hands.

Action
1. Raise your head and shoulders approximately 5 inches (12cms) from the floor.
2. Hold the position, count to three, and then lower your head and shoulders slowly.
3. Do between 6 and 12 reps per set.

Notice!
1. When your raise you head and shoulders, try and keep your elbows back.
2. Try not to move your legs. Keep them over your hips when you're doing this exercise.

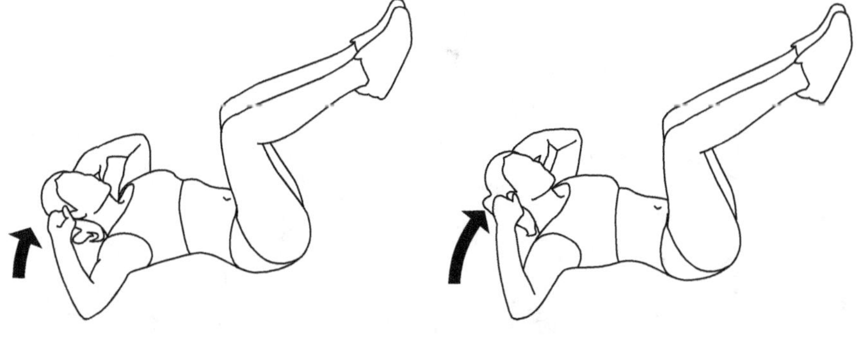

Exercise 10
ABDOMINALS – LOWER

Begin
1. Lie flat on the floor.
2. Put your arms down by your side, palms flat on the floor.
3. Lift your legs, keeping your feet together so that your knees are just above your hips.

Action
1. Lift your hips off the floor, curling your lower body up towards your chest. Your hips should be approximately 4 inches (10cms) off the floor.
2. Hold this position, count to three, then slowly lower your hips.
3. Do between 6 and 12 reps per set.

Notice!
1. Keep your palms flat against the floor.
2. Breathe out as you raise your hips.
3. Don't jerk your hips off the ground. It should be a smooth, gradual movement.

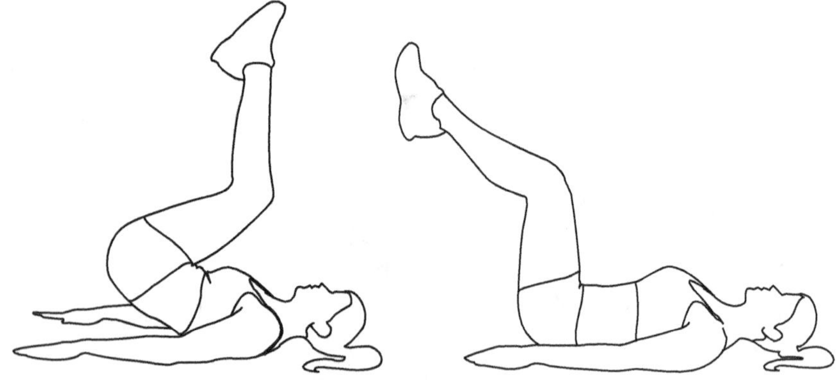

Exercise 11
BACK AND BUTTOCKS

Begin
1. Lie face down on the floor.
2. Place your hands either side of your head as if you were saluting with both hands, elbows out to the side.

Action
1. Raise your head, chest and shoulders from the floor. Exhale.
2. Hold the position and count to three. Breathe normally.
3. Slowly lower yourself to the starting position. Inhale.
4. Do between 5 and 10 reps per set.

Notice!
1. Keep your legs straight and together.
2. Don't jerk yourself off the floor. Use a smooth, controlled movement. Don't overstretch.

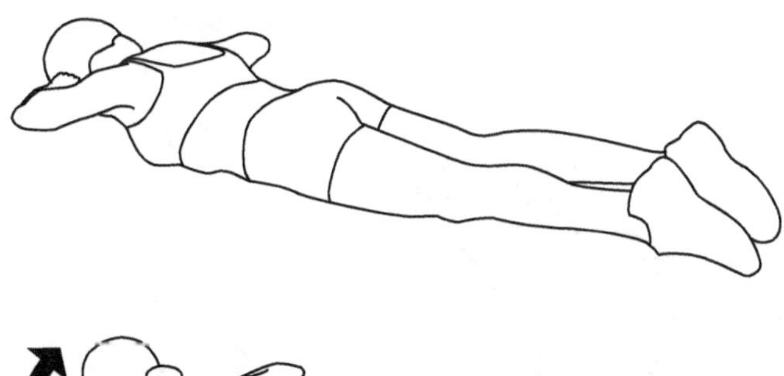

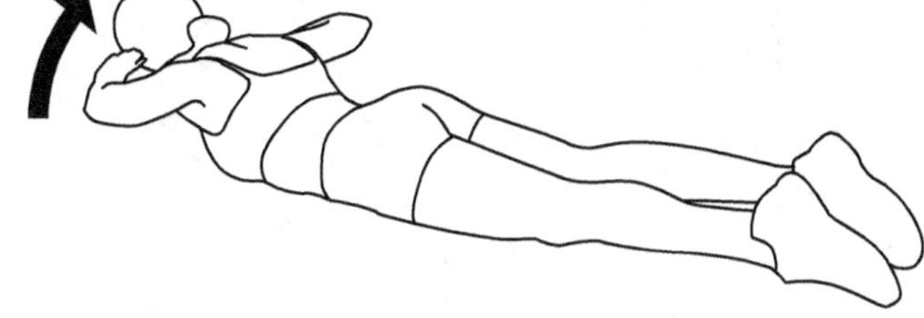

Exercise 12
BACK AND BUTTOCKS

Begin
1. Lie face down on the floor, legs very slightly apart.
2. Stretch your arms out in front of you, palms facing downwards.

Action
1. Raise your left arm and your right leg at the same time.
2. Hold the position and count to three.
3. Do the same, this time using your right arm and left leg.
4. Do 6–12 reps per set.

Notice!
1. Try and keep your head down.
2. Don't overstretch.

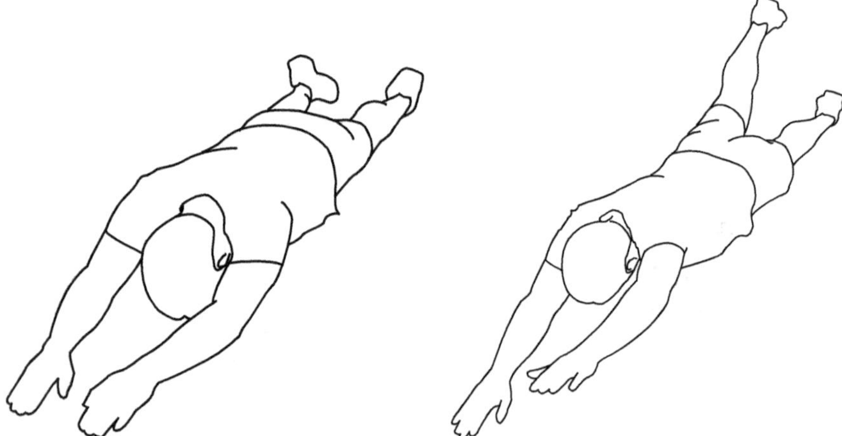

Flexibility exercise

When you take aerobic and resistance exercise your muscles get stronger, but they also get stiffer and tighter. They lose some of their elasticity. The way to get over this is to do *flexibility exercises*. This will stretch your muscles and keep them supple. It will help you to function better.

Flexibility exercise will increase your co-ordination and help to lubricate your joints, as well as increasing the circulation of blood and reducing muscle ache.

Before you start flexibility exercises

You won't lose weight by doing flexibility exercises, but they'll help you reach a new level of fitness by stretching the muscles you use in your aerobic and resistance exercises, and keeping them supple. These exercises are important because they keep your joints flexible and stable, and they reduce the risk of injury. Stretching and flexing your muscles and joints also makes you feel better. Try to do stretching exercises *before* and *after* you take exercise.

Technique

When you start to stretch, you should always do so slowly and gradually. You should be able to feel a gradual pulling on your muscles. Don't lock your joints when you are stretching, and whatever you do, don't bounce or jerk or you will cause injury. Breathe in as you begin to stretch, and as you relax and let go, breathe out. Don't immediately go into another stretch after you've completed one. Take a few seconds out, and then start again.

Useful tips

- When you stretch, concentrate on the muscle you are stretching.
- Don't bounce. Stretch gradually.
- Stretch until you feel slight tension in the muscle.
- Hold the stretch for about 10 – 15 seconds.
- If the tension increases while you are holding the stretch, or you feel pain, release the tension. If muscles feel they are being over-stretched, they will contract to protect themselves.
- Don't hold your breath when you stretch. Breathe normally.
- If you're stressed, stretching will help. Stretching your muscles helps to release tension.
- Before you go to bed, have a good stretch. You'll sleep so much better. Take a hint from animals – they have a good stretch before they sleep.

EXERCISES

Here are a series of eighteen flexibility exercises or 'stretches'. Spend at least 5 minutes every day doing stretching exercises. Vary the ones you do.

Spend 5 minutes every day doing stretching exercises!

Stretch 1
Extend your arms above your head, and intertwine your fingers, your palms facing upward. Stretch your arms upwards and feel the stretch in your outer arms, your shoulders and your ribs.

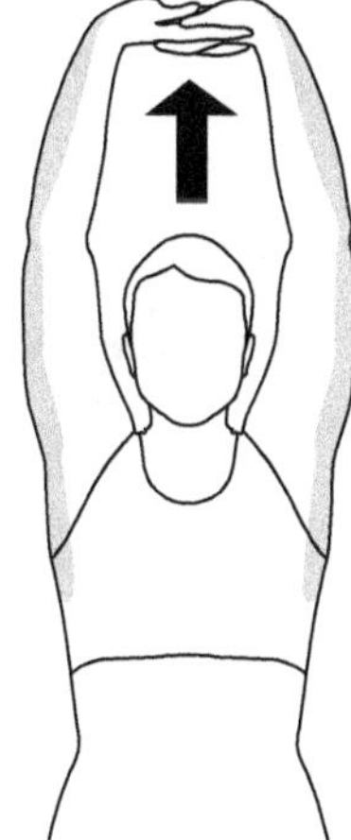

Stretch 2
Extend your arms in front of you and intertwine your fingers, palms facing forward. Push forwards and feel the stretch in your arms and shoulders.

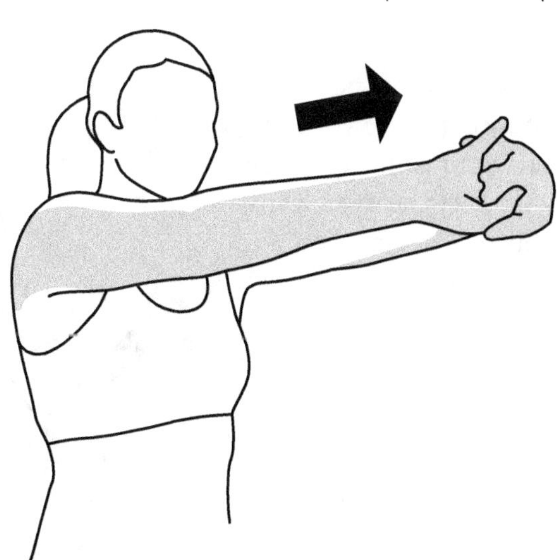

Stretch 3

Raise your shoulders towards your ears, as if you were shrugging. Feel the stretch in your neck and shoulders.

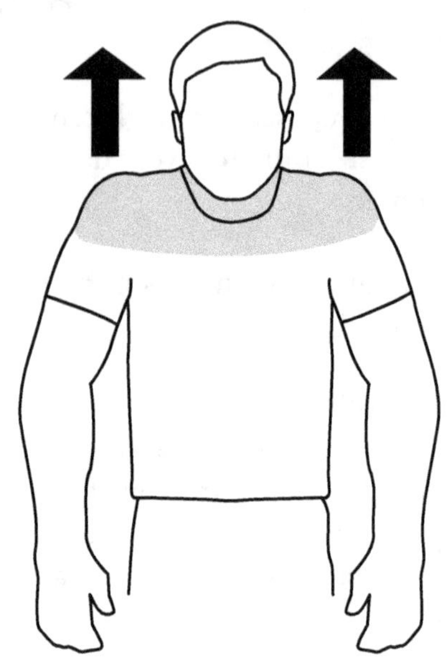

Stretch 4

Put your arms behind you and intertwine your fingers. Lift your arms up behind you. Feel the stretch in your top arms, chest and shoulders.

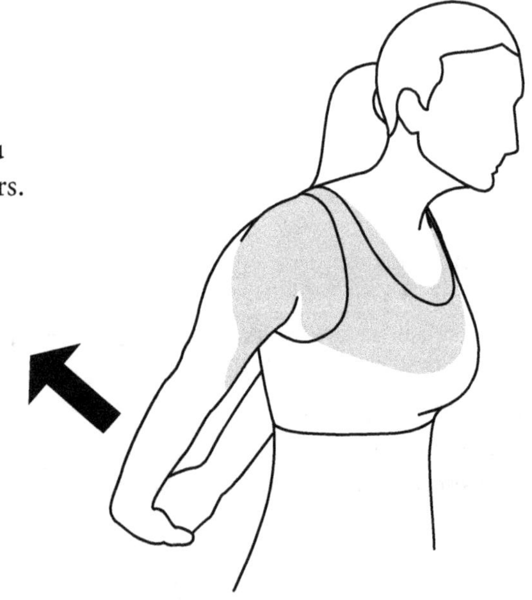

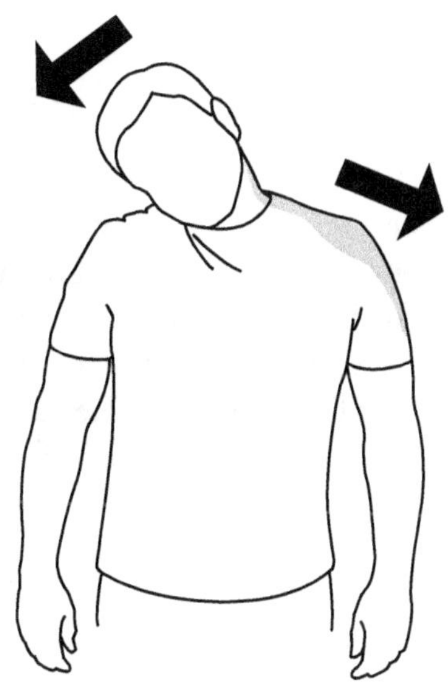

Stretch 5

Lean your head to one side and at the same time lower your shoulder. Feel the stretch in your neck and shoulder. Repeat the stretch on the other side, slowly and carefully.

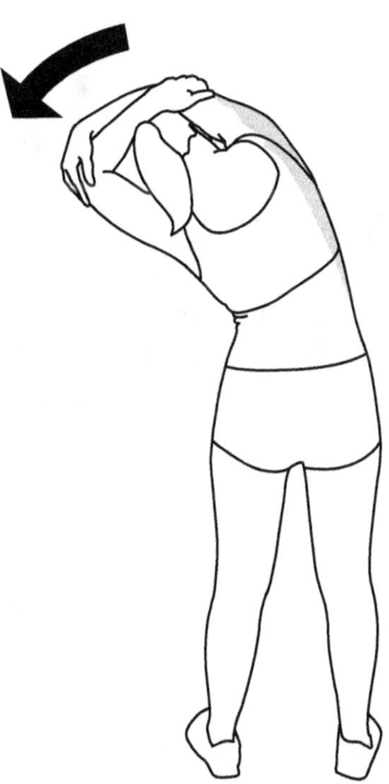

Stretch 6

With your feet apart and your knees not locked, put your left arm behind your head and grasp your left elbow with your right hand. Bend your body to the right until you feel resistance. Feel the stretch on the back of your upper arm and down the left side of your trunk. Repeat the stretch on the other side, this time grasping your right elbow with your left hand.

Stretch 7

With your legs slightly apart, knees slightly bent, your feet pointing forward and your hands on your hips, rotate your hips to the right and look over your right shoulder. Feel the stretch in your lower back and hips. Repeat on the left side. Do two or three repetitions of this stretch.

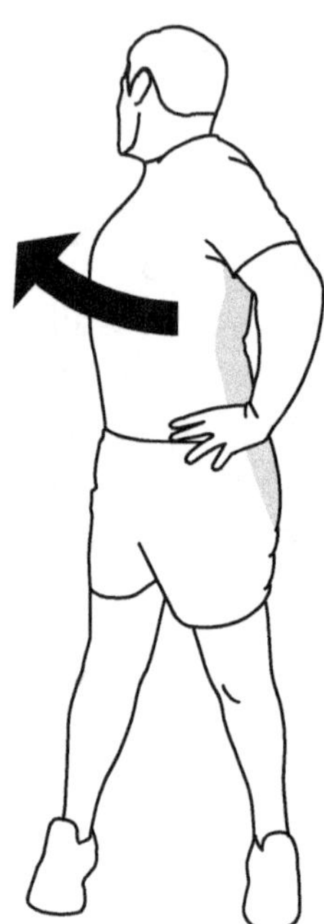

Stretch 8

Place your feet facing forwards and your legs apart. Put your hands on your lower back just behind your hips. Push your lower back forward and keep your elbows back. Feel the stretch in your shoulders, chest and the of top of your arms.

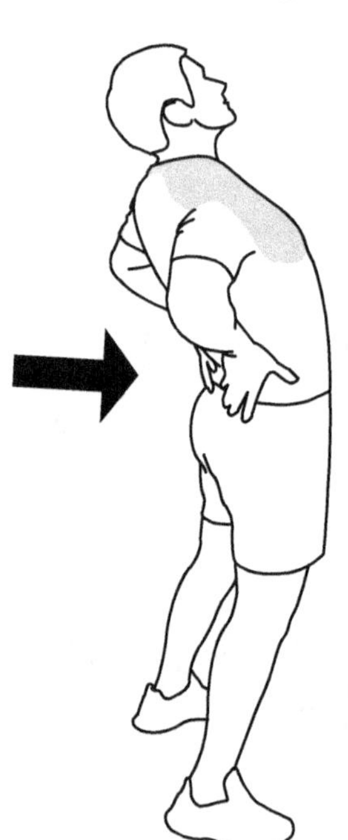

Stretch 9

Stand up straight with your feet pointing forward and your knees slightly bent. Always keep your knees slightly bent during this stretch. Bend forward from your hips and let your arms hang down in front of you. If you can't touch the floor, just let the weight of your body pull you towards the floor. Don't bounce when you do this stretch. Hold the position for 10 – 15 seconds, and then slowly stand upright again. Repeat the stretch. Feel the stretch in your lower back, in your gluteus maximus (your buttocks), and in your hamstrings.

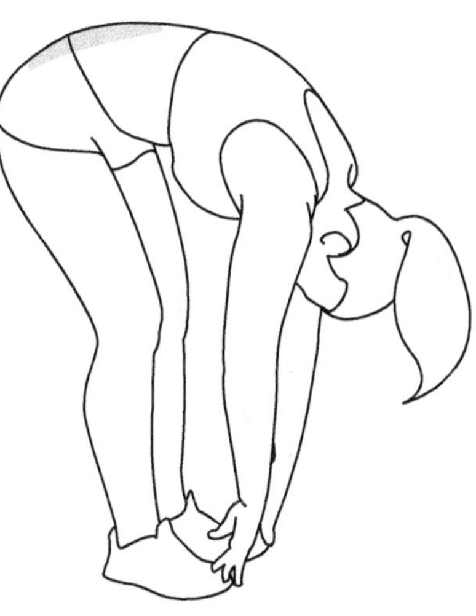

Stretch 10

Stand in front of a wall. Put one hand on the wall for support and then lift your right leg up behind you and hold with your left hand. Pull your foot gently towards your bottom. Feel the stretch in your quads (top front leg) your front lower leg, your knee, and the top of your foot. Repeat the stretch with the other leg.

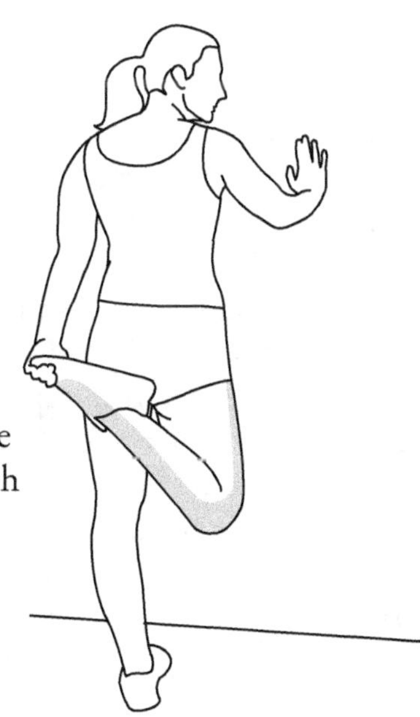

Stretch 11

Stand at arms' length in front of a wall. Bend one leg and place one foot approximately 18 inches (45cms) behind you. Keep your feet flat on the floor. Do not bounce! Gently push your hips gently forward. Feel the stretch in your calf and the top of your foot. Repeat with the other leg.

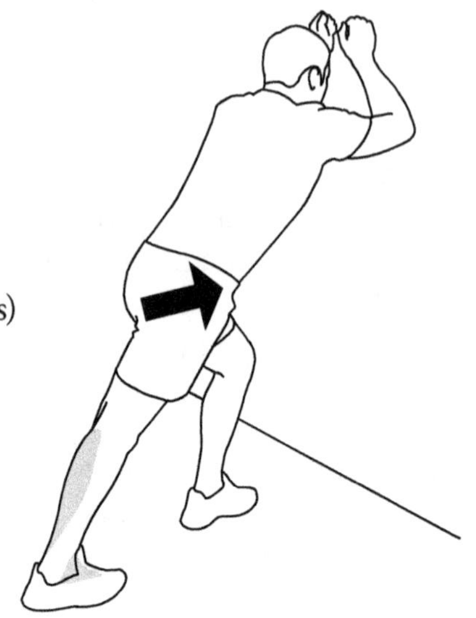

Stretch 12

Kneel down. Lift one knee so that the top of your leg is parallel to the ground. Put both hands on your knee and keep your balance. Slide your other knee backwards, keeping the top of your foot in contact with the ground. Keep upright and lower your hips. Feel the stretch in the groin, the hamstring and the hip. Repeat with the other leg.

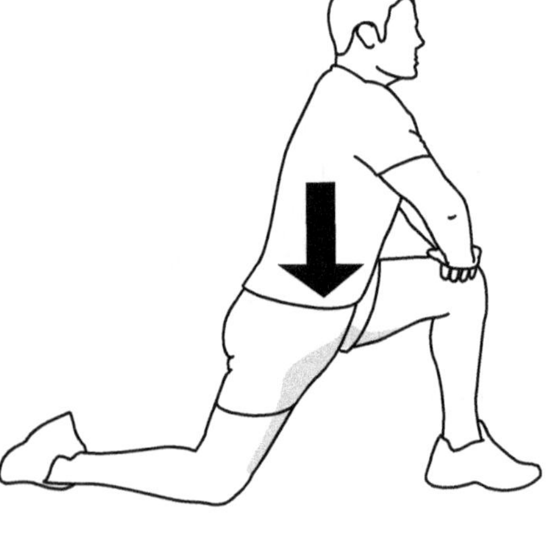

Stretch 13

Lie down on your back. Lift one leg and place your hands in front of your knee. Keep your head in contact with the floor. Pull your leg towards your chest. Feel the stretch in your lower back, hamstring and knee.

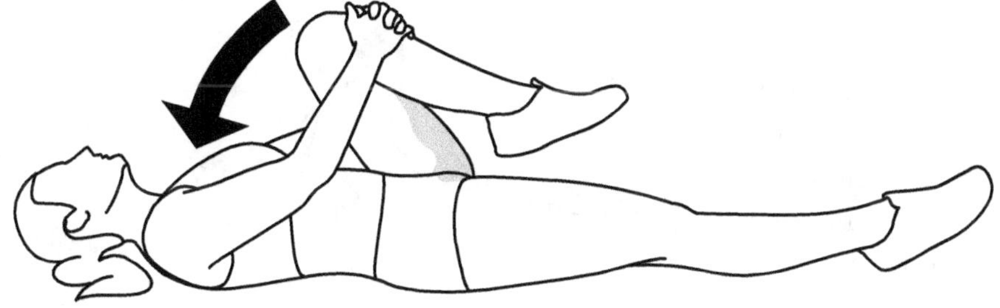

Stretch 14

Sit on the floor. Spread your legs to the sides and then pull your feet towards you. Holding on to your feet, bend forward and gently pull yourself forward. Feel the stretch in your groin and your back.

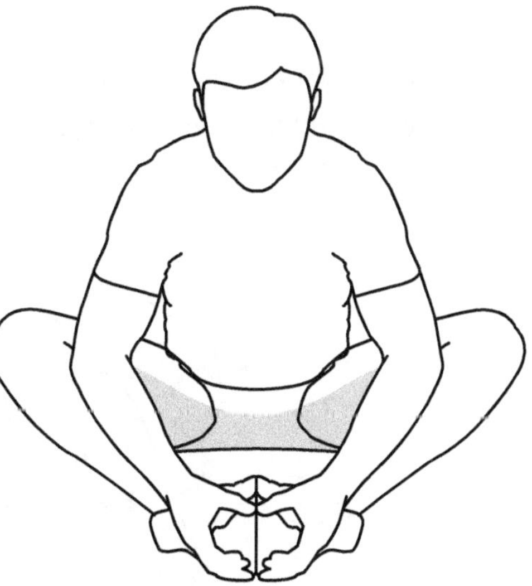

Stretch 15

Sit on the floor. Lift your left leg and cross it over the other leg, so that your foot is beside your right knee. Bend your right elbow and rest against your left knee. Put your right hand behind you, and rotate your upper body towards your left arm. Repeat with the other leg. Feel the stretch in your ribs, upper and lower back and hips. This exercise needs to be done slowly and carefully.

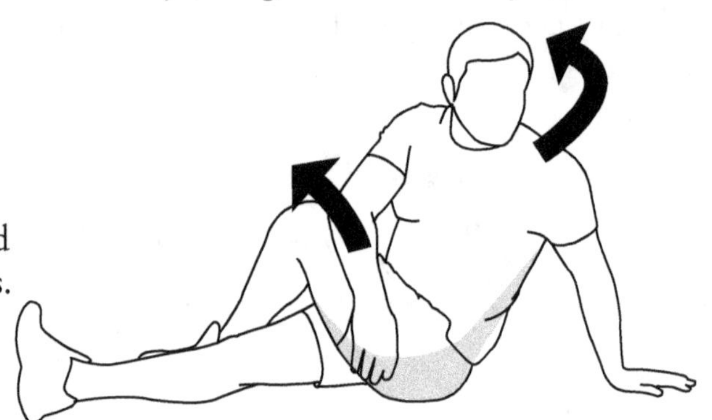

Stretch 16

Lie on the floor, knees bent and feet apart. Put your hands behind your head and intertwine your fingers. Slowly pull your head forwards. Feel the stretch in your neck and spine.

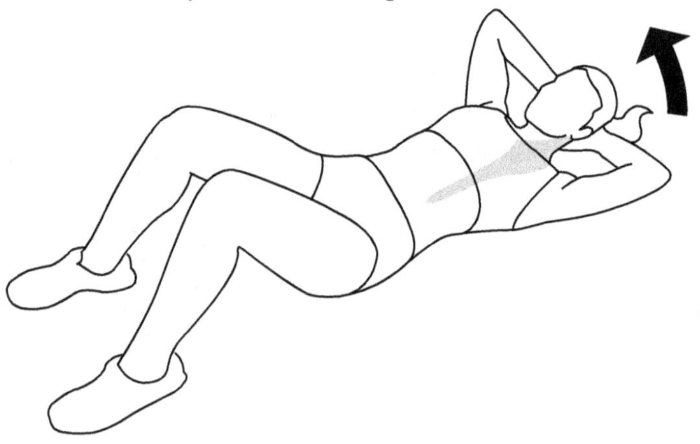

Stretch 17

Kneel on the floor. Lower your head, stretch your arms in front of you, and place your palms flat on the floor. Stretch forward and then pull back pressing your palms down at the same time. Feel the stretch in your shoulders, arms, down the side of your body, and your upper back.

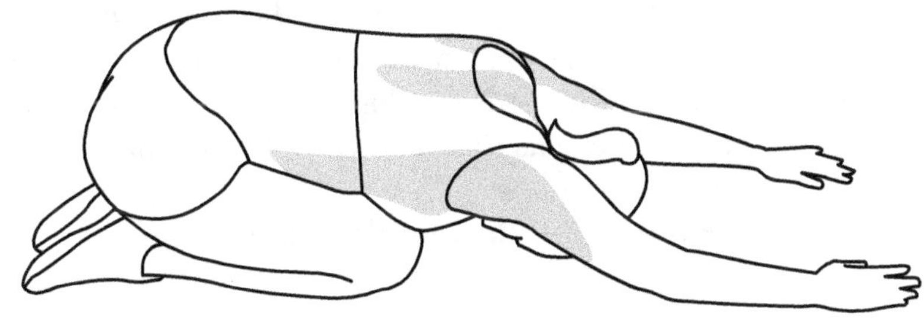

Stretch 18

Lie flat on your back on the floor. Place your arms on the floor behind your head. Now point your toes and point your fingers. Reach out and point as far as you can, and then relax. Now point your right leg and your left arm. Then your left leg and your right arm. Repeat. Feel the stretch in your abdominal muscles, your spine, your shoulders, arms, legs and feet.

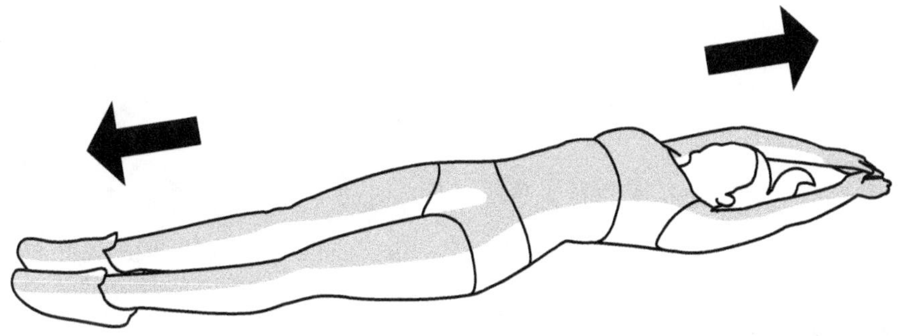

Your opportunity

The benefit of learning new habits is that they replace old habits. They become an established part of what you do, part of your routine, part of your life. Unlike a diet, they have lasting benefits.

You now have the key to a slim, healthy life: the knowledge and the means to manage your weight and to stay slim and healthy, and a foundation on which to make improvements to your diet and to your exercise regime. Continuous improvement should be your aim, whether it is discovering new, healthy foods or adopting a more adventurous, fun way to exercise. The benefits that follow will be life-changing.

Enjoy your slim healthy life

Low Calorie Day menus

Low Calorie Day total calorie allowance: **550 calories**

Here are a some simple rules about Low Calorie days to help you:

1. Always include protein in your breakfast meal. It takes longer to metabolize protein and this will make you feel less hungry.

2. Work out the calorie values and the quantities of your Low Calorie Day menus in advance.

3. **Simple is best. It's not recommended that you spend time thinking about food or preparing mouthwatering culinary masterpieces on Low Calorie Days.**

4. If you feel hungry between meals, drink a glass of water.

5. Try and eat your last meal of the day as early as possible. Twelve hours between your evening meal and breakfast next day is good.

There are lots of websites that will give you ideas for your Low Calorie Day meals. A good piece of advice for Low Calorie Days is **'don't make a meal out of your meals'**. Below are a list of ingredients and some suggestions for some simple meals. Make up your own menu plans and keep them simple and easy to prepare.

Breakfast

We all tend to eat the same sort of thing every day for breakfast. Do the same on Low Calorie Days except make sure you include protein, carbohydrate and fibre. You don't have to eat lots of calories to have a good breakfast. Here are a list of options. Mix and match them to suit your preferences.

Protein:

Egg, fried, boiled, poached, scrambled, coddled	**80kcal**
Ham, slice	**37kcal**
Cheese cheddar small slice	**113kcal**
Plain fat-free yogurt 50g	**28kcal**

Fruit: (for fibre)

Banana	**48kcal**
Blueberries (25)	**19kcal**
Pear	**45kcal**
Apple	**48kcal**
Strawberries (6)	**13kcal**
Raspberries (20)	**20kcal**
Peach	**51kcal**

Carbohydrate: (Cereal)

Muesli ¼ cup/25g	**91kcal**
All-Bran ½ cup/50g	**80kcal**
Special K ½ cup/50g	**60kcal**
Porridge 1 × serving	**160kcal**
1 serving skimmed milk (for cereal)	**15kcal**

Carbohydrate (other)

Slice wholemeal toast	**75kcal**
Bagel	**69kcal**
(1 × small pat of butter)	**36kcal**

Drink:

Coffee with skimmed milk	**15kcal**
Tea with skimmed milk	**7kcal**
Green tea	**0kcal**

Here are three breakfast combinations:

Option 1

Fried egg on toast (with butter)	**191kcal**
Half a banana	**24kcal**
1 cup of tea with skimmed milk	**7kcal**
Total kcal	**222kcal**

Option 2

Special K and skimmed milk	**75kcal**
Strawberries	**13kcal**
Boiled egg	**80kcal**
1 cup of coffee with skimmed milk	**15kcal**
Total kcal	**183kcal**

Option 3

Poached egg on toast with ham	**192kcal**
½ apple	**24kcal**
1 cup of green tea	**0kcal**
Total kca	**216kcal**

Easy lunch and evening meals

If you work and you normally buy your lunch, you may find it difficult to keep within your calorie limits because you're dealing with small numbers. The calories on some over-the-counter foods might be difficult to identify. To get round this you might decide it's easier to prepare your lunch and take it with you. Vegetable dishes, including salads, are low in calories and can be filling – especially if you include protein.

The following list of ingredients can be used to make lots of different simple dishes which can be your lunch or evening meal. Homemade soup is always a useful thing to have in the fridge. Be careful of bought soups – particularly tinned soups – as many are high in calories and contain a lot of salt and sugar. Miso soup, which comes in small sachets, is very low in calories (40kcal) and is great for Low Calorie Days or for your lunch or evening meal.

Be aware of the portion sizes of the ingredients listed. **They are small portions**. Weigh out some of the ingredients to make sure you know what 30g of French beans looks like, for example.

Protein

Beef, sliced 30g	60kcal
Beef minced/ground 30g	65kcal
Cannellini beans 40g	34kcal
Chicken breast (small w/o skin)	124kcal
Chicken thigh (small w/o skin)	82kcal
Cottage Cheese 30g	27kcal
Egg	80kcal
Ham, slice	37kcal
Hummus 20g	33kcal
Lentils 30	35kcal
Mozzarella cheese – ¼ cheese	80kcal
Pork/Beef sausage	81kcal
Prawns /shrimps 30g	90kcal
Sardines tinned 40g	83kcal
Tofu 50g	50kcal
Tuna tinned 60g	70kcal

Carbohydrates

Brown rice 30g	35kcal
Cauliflower 70g	16kcal
Couscous 40g	45kcal
New potatoes 70g	60kcal
Rye bread, one slice	83kcal
Wholemeal bread, one slice	75kcal
Wholewheat pasta 40g	50kcal
Bean sprouts 30g	9kcal

Broccoli 50g — **18kcal**
Cabbage 50g — **11kcal**
Carrots 30g — **12kcal**
Celery 30g — **4kcal**
French beans 40g — **7kcal**
Lettuce 30g — **5kcal**
Mushrooms 25g — **6kcal**
Onion 50g — **21kcal**
Pak choi 50g — **7kcal**
Peas 30g — **23kcal**
Red pepper (1) — **30kcal**
Salad, mixed one serving — **17kcal**
Spring onion (3) — **5kcal**
Sweet corn 30g — **24kcal**
Tomatoes, cherry (5) — **25kcal**
Zucchini / courgette (small) — **20kcal**

Other

Cheese sauce, 5 tablespoons — **124kcal**
Macaroni /pasta 70g — **111kcal**
Miso soup, sachet — **40kcal**
Olive oil, tablespoon — **135kcal**
Pesto, 1 tablespoon — **39kcal**

Here are some lunch and evening meal suggestions.
Portion sizes are important. Keep them small, to the recommended size.

Omelette

Omelettes are simple and easy to do:
2 eggs — **160kcal**
Small mixed salad — **17kcal**
Total — **177kcal**

Add other ingredients to make your omelette more interesting:
Mushrooms, cheese or ham and add the additional calories to the total.

Salads

Easy to prepare, salads are a great Low Calorie Day food.

Small mixed salad	17kcal
Small mixed salad with 2 slices of ham & French beans	98kcal
Small mixed salad with chicken breast & brown rice	176kcal
Small mixed salad with cottage cheese & egg	124kcal
Small mixed salad with tuna and tomato	112kcal
Small mixed salad with egg & ham	134kcal
Small mixed salad with tofu and couscous	112kcal
Small mixed salad with prawns & brown rice	142kcal

Bean salad

Cannellini beans, cooked French beans, celery, Spring onion, tomato, olive oil	210kcal

'On toast'

Scrambled/poached egg on toast with butter	191kcal
Sardines on toast with butter	194kcal
Avocado and tomato on toast with butter	176kcal
Mushrooms on toast with butter	118kcal

Other suggestions

Cauliflower 70g, cheese sauce, 5 tablespoons	140kcal
Macaroni 70g, cheese sauce, 5 tablespoons	235kcal
Pasta 70g, olive oil 1 tablespoon	246kcal
Pasta 70g, pesto 1 tablespoon	150kcal
Brown rice 30g, prawns 30g, bean sprouts 30g, peas 30g	157kcal

Keep your Low Calorie Day menus simple and easy to prepare. Draw up a list of meal options you can refer to so you don't have to spend lots of time thinking about food or its preparation.

References

World Health Organisation: Fact Sheet #311 'Obesity and Overweight' 2015

'Childhood Overweight and Obesity' World Health Organisation 2014

'Adult Obesity and Type 2 Diabetes' Public Health England 2014

'Changing the Future of Obesity' www.ncbi.ntm.gov/pm/articles

Krebs: 'The Gourmet Ape: Evolution and Human Food Preferences' American Society for Nutrition

'Developmental and epigenetic pathways to obesity: an evolutionary-developmental perspective' P D Gluckman, M A Hanson *International Journal of Obesity*

'Nutrition and Evolution' by Michael Crawford and David Marsh.

'Origins and evolution of the Western diet: health implications for the 21st century' Cordain, Boyd Eaton *et al*

'Relationship between stress, eating behavior, and obesity' *Science Direct* Susan Torres and Caryl Nowson

'The link between stress and obesity' D.Thompson www.everyday-health .com

'Lifetime Health and Economic Consequences of Obesity' D. Thompson et al

'The Skinny on Obesity' Dr Robert Lustig UCTV Prime

'Hunger and Eating' Takako Hara California State University 1997

'How Fat Cells Work' C Freudenreich

'The Impact of Advertising on Childhood Obesity' American Psychological Association

'Food Advertising and Childhood Obesity' Termini, Roberto, Hostetter. Social Science Research Network 2011

'Cortisol — Its Role in Stress, Inflammation, and Indications for Diet Therapy' Dina Aronson: *Today's Dietician*

'Fat Chance' Dr Robert Lustig 33–47, 49–50, 52–53, 66–71, 81–84, 117–138

'Obesity, Leptin resistance, and the Effects of Insulin': International Journal of Obesity; Lustig, Sen, Soberman, Valasquez-Mieyer

'Health Risks and Disease: Salt and sodium': T H Chan, School of Public Health

'Is Obesity an Addiction'; P J Kenny 2013, *Scientific American*

'The impact of water intake on energy intake and weight status' M C Daniels, B M Popkin, US National Library of Health

'Waking Up to Sleep's Role in Weight Control" Harvard, T H Chan, School of Public Health

'Obesity and Alcohol' National Obesity Observatory 2012

'How Artificial Sweeteners Confuse Your Body into Storing Fat and Inducing Diabetes' *Mercola 2014*

'The Toxic Truth About Sugar': R H Lustig, L A Schmidt, Claire D Brindis

'Reward Mechanisms in Obesity: New Insights and Future Directions' Paul J Kenny

'Leptin and Leptin Resistance' Kris Gunnars

'The effect of dietary fiber and other factors on insulin response: role in obesity' I H Ullrich, M J Albrink

'Still Believe "A Calorie Is a Calorie?"' Robert Lustig

'Why fasting boosts your brain power' Mark Mattson, John Hopkins TEDx

Index

About the author

John McPhie has always had a passion for discovering ways of removing obstacles which limit human potential, and for finding simple solutions to complex problems. In a world burdened by an obesity epidemic, where those in need of an answer to their weight problems have been ill-served by diet fads and quick fixes, his prime motivation has been to reveal the true facts, simply and clearly, about why people put on weight. The Slim Habit, developed over several 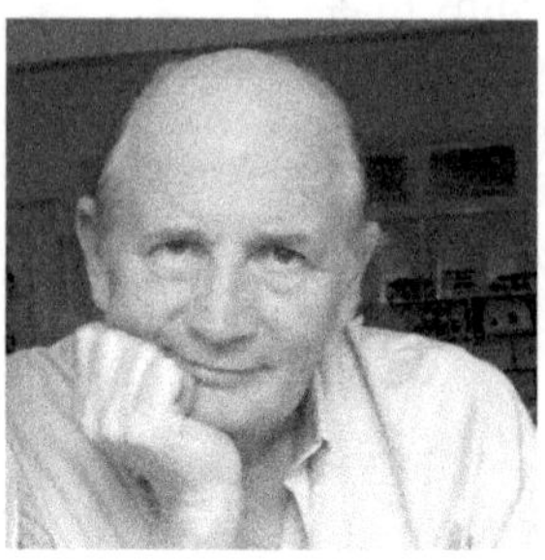
years, incorporates his experience in behavioural science and the very latest medical thinking. The aim of the book is to offer a better understanding about exactly why weight gain happens, and to provide an easy-to-do way of losing it – permanently. The Slim Habit fulfils his ambition to provide a solution that he believes will make a real and lasting difference to peoples' lives.

"Communication is the way to improve the world's health ... spread the word!"

Professor Mark Mattson

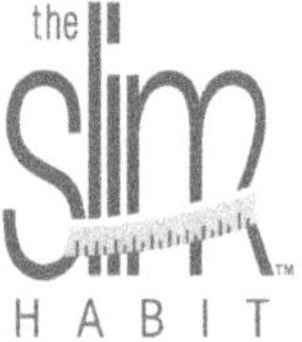
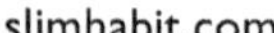
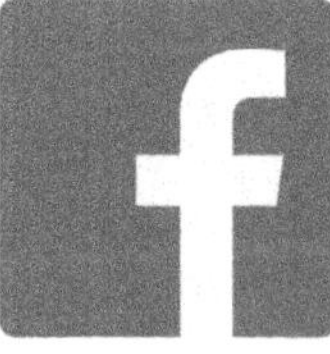
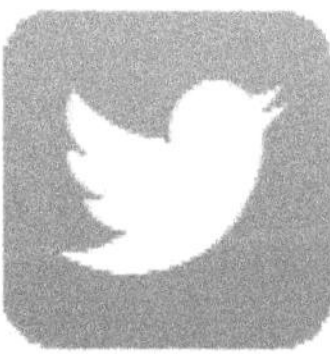

slimhabit.com   Slim-Habit   @slimhabit   /slimhabit/